T0341232

Multiphysics Modeling with Application to Biomedical Engineering

Multiphysics Modeling with Application to Biomedical Engineering

Z. Yang

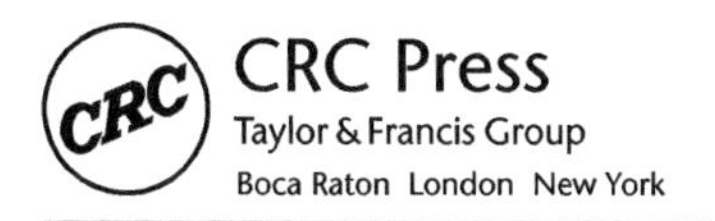

CRC Press is an imprint of the
Taylor & Francis Group, an **informa** business

First edition published 2021
by CRC Press
6000 Broken Sound Parkway NW, Suite 300, Boca Raton, FL 33487-2742

and by CRC Press
2 Park Square, Milton Park, Abingdon, Oxon, OX14 4RN

CRC Press is an imprint of Taylor & Francis Group, LLC

Library of Congress Cataloging-in-Publication Data

Names: Yang, Z., author.
Title: Multiphysics modeling with application to biomedical engineering / Z. Yang.
Description: Boca Raton : CRC Press, 2021. | Includes bibliographical references and index. | Summary: "The aim of this book is to introduce the simulation of various physical fields and their applications for biomedical engineering, which will provide a base for researchers in the biomedical field to conduct further investigation. The entire book is classified into three levels. It starts with the first level, which presents the single physical fields including structural analysis, fluid simulation, thermal analysis, and acoustic modeling. Then, the second level consists of various couplings between two physical fields covering structural thermal coupling, porous media, fluid structural interaction (FSI), and acoustic FSI. The third level focuses on multi-coupling that coupling with more than two physical fields in the model. Each part in all levels is organized as the physical feature, finite element implementation, modeling procedure in ANSYS, and the specific applications for biomedical engineering like the FSI study of Abdominal Aortic Aneurysm (AAA), acoustic wave transmission in the ear, and heat generation of the breast tumor. The book should help for the researchers and graduate students conduct numerical simulation of various biomedical coupling problems. It should also provide all readers with a better understanding of various couplings"-- Provided by publisher.
Identifiers: LCCN 2020009270 (print) | LCCN 2020009271 (ebook) | ISBN 9780367509767 (hardback) | ISBN 9780367510800 (ebook)
Subjects: MESH: Physical Phenomena | Biomedical Engineering | Finite Element Analysis
Classification: LCC R857.M3 (print) | LCC R857.M3 (ebook) | NLM QT 36 | DDC 610.28--dc23
LC record available at https://lccn.loc.gov/2020009270
LC ebook record available at https://lccn.loc.gov/2020009271

ISBN: 978-0-367-50976-7 (hbk)
ISBN: 978-0-367-51080-0 (ebk)

Typeset in Times
by Lumina Datamatics Limited

Contents

SECTION III Coupling among More Than Two Physics Phases

SECTION IV Retrospective

Preface

In 2002, when I started my PhD research at the University of Pittsburgh, my advisor, Dr. Patrick Smolinski, asked me to develop the finite element program to simulate soft tissues in the dynamic state, which incorporates the coupling of solid and fluid phases, large deformation, and viscoelasticity of soft tissues. This request began my research in the field of multiphysics. After my graduation, I worked with Dr. Smolinski on a DOE project to simulate the gas flow in the gas reservoir. For the past twelve years, I have been working in the research & development department in big companies; I have gained significant experiences in the area of finite element development and application, especially the application of multiphysics for biomedical engineering. This book reflects my understanding of coupling simulation that paves a path for the biomedical researchers to conduct further studies. Since the coupling problems involving different physics fields are very complicated, some errors may exist in the book. I ask the readers to point out the errors so that I can correct them.

During the writing and publication of the book, many individuals, including Dr. Patrick Smolinski, Dr. Jeen-Shang Lin, Frank Marx, Dr. Zhi-Hong Mao, Dr. Li Zhao, Dr. Krystyna Gielo-Perczak, and Ronna Edelstein, have helped me deal with various challenges and obstacles. I deeply appreciate their encouragement and assistance. I am also grateful to the CRC Press staff, especially Marc Gutierrez and Nick Mould, for their hard work. Finally, I thank my wife and my two children for their constant patience and support.

Author

Z. Yang obtained his PhD degree in mechanical engineering from the University of Pittsburgh in 2004. Since 2001, he has been engaged in the field of finite element analysis for more than 18 years and has completed many projects in both academia and industry. So far, he has published 30 papers in refereed journals and conference proceedings, including two books (*Finite Element Analysis for Biomedical Engineering Applications* and *Material Modeling in Finite Element Analysis*) by CRC Press.

1 Introduction

Various physical phenomena exist in the human body: cartilages contacting meniscus in the knee; blood flowing in the vessel; air going in and out of the lung; acoustic wave transiting in the ear; and muscle becoming warm after cyclic tension. Clinical studies have found that some diseases have a close association with physical phenomena. Knee pain is linked with the contact pressures in the knee, and back pain is probably caused by the big mechanical loads on the spine. Abdominal aortic aneurysm is a condition in which the terminal aorta deforms to dangerous proportions under blood pressure. The blasts in a military battle often cause tympanic membrane injuries of the ear. Because these diseases are very common—millions of people are struggling with them—great effort has been taken to study them. One of the keys to ending these diseases is to understand the physical states, including stress and deformation of structure, acoustic pressure in the acoustic problems, temperature in the thermal problems, and velocity and pressure in the fluid field. Many studies have addressed these issues by experimental study and numerical simulation. This book focuses on numerical simulation, covering structural analysis, thermal analysis, fluid analysis, and acoustic analysis, and their couplings, such as fluid structural interaction (FSI), porous media, acoustic FSI, and thermal structural coupling.

Recently, numerical simulation has been extensively applied in the fields of academic research and industry. To meet this rising use of numerical simulation, a great deal of commercial software, including ANSYS, Marc, ABAQUS, and Nastran has been developed in the last 50 years. Among them, ANSYS Fluent is the most widely used computational fluid dynamics software, and mechanical analysis in ANSYS is very powerful in structural/thermal/acoustic analysis. Thus, all examples in this book are implemented in ANSYS, and all input files are attached in the appendixes.

The book is divided into four parts. The first part focuses on single physics phases. After Chapter 1 introduces the subject, Chapter 2 describes the structural analysis. It starts with the nature of solid and the Lagrangian description. This is followed by the equilibrium equation and the corresponding finite element matrix form, as well as the modeling procedure in ANSYS. Chapter 2 ends with a simulation of the deformation of the intervertebral disc under pressure.

Fluid dynamics is briefly discussed in Chapter 3. Because fluid flows freely under loading, the Eulerian description is applied for the fluid field. After describing the governing equations and general modeling procedure in ANSYS Fluent, the blood flow through a stenotic artery is simulated in ANSYS Fluent.

Chapter 4 introduces acoustics, including its wave characteristics, the wave governing equation and corresponding finite element matrix form, and harmonic analysis of a body under a blast in the open area.

Thermal analysis is the focus of Chapter 5. After introducing the governing equation and finite element matrix form, as well as the finite element procedure of the thermal analysis, the heat generation of the breast tumor is modeled and verified by the reference results.

Part I introduces the single physics fields, and Part II turns to the couplings between them. After a short introduction of the general coupling methods and classification in Chapter 6, Chapter 7 presents FSI and its simulation procedure in ANSYS. In the last part of Chapter 7, a FSI study of abdominal aortic aneurysm is performed by two-way coupling and one-way coupling, and then compared against the results of the static analysis.

Biological soft tissues are biphasic with the coupling of the solid and fluid phases, which can be modeled by coupled pore-pressure thermal (CPT) elements in ANSYS. Chapter 8 introduces the governing equations and general modeling procedure of CPT elements. Then, it shows a simulation of biological tissues in the confined compression test.

Compared with FSI, acoustic FSI is relatively simple due to the linear acoustic governing equations. After listing the governing equations and simulation procedure in ANSYS in the first two parts of Chapter 9, the acoustic wave transmission in the ear is studied using acoustic FSI.

Chapter 10 presents the thermal structural analysis, which starts with thermal-structural coupling equations and modeling procedures in ANSYS, and it follows the study of temperature change of biological tissues under cycle loadings.

Part III discusses models with more than two physical fields. With more physical fields, the coupling problems become more complicated, and it is more difficult to reach convergence. Two cases are presented in Chapters 11 and 12, respectively. Chapter 11 focuses on the thermal problem of soft tissues, in which the thermal analysis works with CPT elements. The thermal analysis of porous media is implemented in ANSYS using CPT elements with keyopt(11) = 1 and applied for modeling the tissue fusion in the last part of Chapter 11. Another case in Chapter 12 studies the murmur detected in the skin surface due to blocking in the blood vessel. This case is solved with two couplings: (1) one coupling between the blood flow and wall of the vessel and (2) another acoustic FSI between the vessel (solid) and the soft tissues (fluid).

The last part is retrospective. Based on the above three parts, Chapter 13 describes the influence of physics natures on physical modeling, problem-dependent coupling methods, special meshing requirements for various physical models, and units for coupling problems.

Multiphysics is a big field. Besides the couplings mentioned in the book, it also includes piezoelectric analysis, electrostatic-structure coupling, magneto-structure coupling, magneto-fluid coupling, electrothermal coupling, and magnetic-thermal coupling. These couplings are not covered in the book because they occur rarely in biomedical engineering. If the readers are interested in these couplings, they may read the relevant part of the ANSYS theory manual and other reference books, such as Chapter 22 in *Material Modeling in Finite Element Analysis* (CRC Press, 2019), Chapter 2 in *Multiphysics Modeling: Numerical Methods and Engineering Applications* (Elsevier, 2015), and *Multiphysics Modeling with Finite Element Methods* (World Scientific Publishing, 2006).

Most examples in the book have been implemented using ANSYS Parametric Design Language. Reading this book requires knowledge of the ANSYS Parametric Design Language. I suggest the readers to study the ANSYS help documentation, and then practice some problems in *Finite Element Analysis for Biomedical Engineering Applications* (CRC Press, 2019).

Section I

Single Physics Phases

The first section focuses on single physics phases, including structural analysis, fluid analysis, thermal analysis, and acoustic analysis. These single physics phases have their unique features and corresponding modeling procedure in ANSYS, which Chapter 2 through Chapter 5 discuss.

Chapter 2 presents structural analysis. After briefly introducing the finite deformation of the solid and the corresponding balance equations, as well as the ANSYS modeling procedure, the intervertebral disc under pressure is simulated in ANSYS.

Fluid analysis is the topic of Chapter 3. Unlike a solid, fluid is easily deformed. The governing equation of the fluid and modeling procedure in ANSYS Fluent are presented along with one example of blood flowing through a stenotic artery.

Sound is a wave controlled by the wave equation. Chapter 4 introduces the governing equation of acoustic, finite element procedure, and its application for studying a body under a blast in an open area.

Heat transfer occurs whenever the temperature gradient exists. The thermal conductivity equation and finite element modeling are discussed in the first section of Chapter 5. That is followed by the thermal analysis of a breast tumor.

2 Structural Analysis

Clinical studies have found that many common diseases are linked to the stress state of the solid phase. For example, knee pain is always associated with the contact pressure of the knee [1], and an extremely high load often causes back pain. Thus, the structural analysis in a biomedical study is receiving more and more attention.

Chapter 2 discusses the nature of the solid state, the governing equation of the solid, and the finite element implementation, and gives one example that models the intervertebral disc under compression.

2.1 GENERAL CHARACTERISTIC OF SOLID STATE

Matter can exist in three states: solid, liquid, and gas. Under a given set of conditions of temperature and pressure, the most stable state of a given substance depends upon the net effect of two opposing factors—intermolecular forces tending to keep the molecules (or atoms or ions) closer and thermal energy tending to keep them apart by making them move faster. At a sufficiently low temperature, the thermal energy is low enough for intermolecular forces to bring the molecules so close that they cling to one another and occupy fixed positions. Because these molecules can still oscillate about their mean positions, the substance exists in a solid state. The solid state has the following characteristic properties [2]:

1. definite mass, volume, and shape;
2. short intermolecular distances;
3. strong intermolecular forces;
4. constituent particles (atoms, molecules, or ions) with fixed positions that can only oscillate about their mean positions; and
5. high stiffness.

2.2 GOVERNING EQUATION OF SOLID AND FINITE ELEMENT IMPLEMENTATION

The solid has a definite shape and undergoes finite deformation under external loadings when the rigid motion is not considered. The finite deformation can be defined by the Lagrangian description [3].

2.2.1 Lagrangian Description

The reference configuration Ω_0 is the configuration occupied by the material at time $t = 0$, which is also called the initial configuration (Figure 2.1). A material point A in the reference configuration is assigned a unique vector $\mathbf{X}$. Later, the material moves to

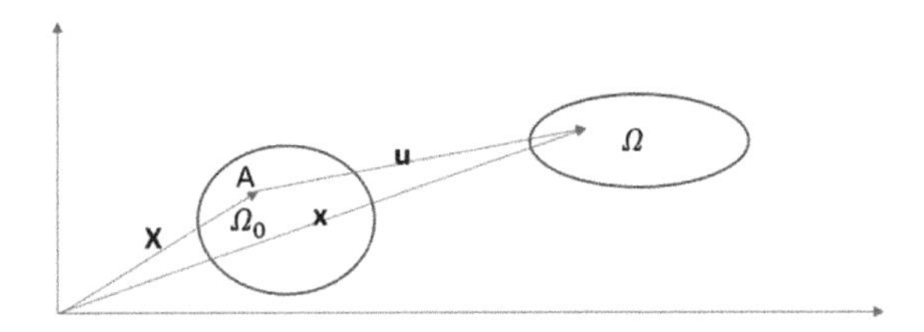

FIGURE 2.1 Lagrangian description.

another configuration (current configuration) Ω. Material point A in the current configuration is then given a new vector **x**. The relation between **X** and **x** can be expressed by:

$$\mathbf{x} = \chi(\mathbf{X}, t) \tag{2.1}$$

The deformation of A is computed by:

$$\mathbf{u} = \mathbf{x} - \mathbf{X} \tag{2.2}$$

The Green strain tensor is written in terms of deformation gradients [3]:

$$\mathbf{e} = \frac{1}{2}\left((\nabla_0\mathbf{u})^{\mathrm{T}} + \nabla_0\mathbf{u} + \nabla_0\mathbf{u}(\nabla_0\mathbf{u})^{\mathrm{T}}\right) \tag{2.3}$$

where ∇_0 is the gradient operator.

In the case of small strains, the term $\nabla_0\mathbf{u}(\nabla_0\mathbf{u})^{\mathrm{T}}$ in the above equation is negligible. The discussions in Section 2.1 are limited to the linear elasticity with small strains. Under such conditions, the elastic strain ε is equal to the total strain **e**.

2.2.2 Constitutive Equation

The constitutive equation is expressed as [3]:

$$\sigma = \mathbf{D} : \varepsilon \tag{2.4}$$

where:

σ = stress;
ε = elastic strain; and
D = the fourth order tensor.

2.2.3 Governing Equations and Boundary Conditions for Structural Analysis

The equilibrium equation can be written as [4]:

$$\nabla \cdot \sigma + \mathbf{b} = \rho \frac{\partial^2 \mathbf{u}}{\partial t^2} \tag{2.5}$$

where:

$\mathbf{b}$ = a force per unit volume and
ρ = mass density.

The boundary conditions include [4]:

$$\mathbf{u} = \bar{\mathbf{u}} \text{ on } S_u \tag{2.6}$$

$$\mathbf{n}\boldsymbol{\sigma} = \bar{\mathbf{t}} \text{ on } S_t \tag{2.7}$$

where:

S_u and S_t = the boundary relevant to the displacements and surface tractions, respectively;
$\mathbf{n}$ = the unit outward normal to the boundary;
$\bar{\mathbf{u}}$ = displacements prescribed on the boundary of S_u; and
$\bar{\mathbf{t}}$ = surface tractions prescribed on the boundary of S_t.

2.2.4 Finite Element Implementation

In the finite element analysis, the continuous body is divided into many elements (Figure 2.2). The principle of virtual work states that the internal virtual work is equal to the external virtual work [3],

$$\int_V \boldsymbol{\sigma}^{\mathrm{T}} \delta \boldsymbol{\varepsilon} dV = \int_{S_t} \bar{\mathbf{t}}^{\mathrm{T}} \delta \mathbf{u} dS + \int_V \bar{\mathbf{b}}^{\mathrm{T}} \delta \mathbf{u} dV \tag{2.8}$$

The displacement of any point in each element can be approximated from the nodes of the element [2]:

$$\mathbf{u}(\mathbf{X},t) = \mathbf{N}(\mathbf{X})\mathbf{u}_e(t) = \sum_I N_I(\mathbf{X}) u_I^e(t) \tag{2.9}$$

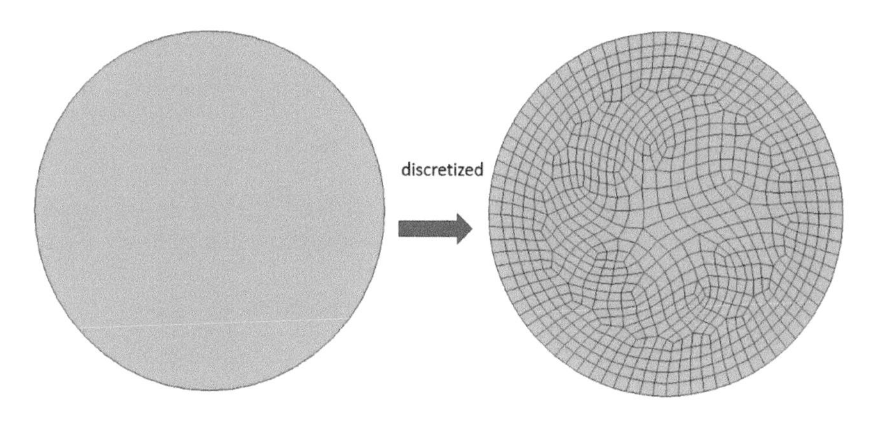

FIGURE 2.2 Discretization of geometry into elements.

Therefore, the strains can be expressed as:

$$\varepsilon = \mathbf{B}\mathbf{u}_e \tag{2.10}$$

where $\mathbf{B} = \partial\mathbf{N}$:

and stresses have the following form:

$$\sigma = \mathbf{D}\mathbf{B}\mathbf{u}_e \tag{2.11}$$

Substituting the above Equations (2.9)–(2.11) into the weak form of the virtual work Equation (2.8), the equilibrium equation in the linear elastic case with small strains can be written into the matrix form as [5]:

$$\mathbf{M}_e^s\ddot{\mathbf{u}}_e + \mathbf{K}_e^s\mathbf{u}_e = \mathbf{f}_e^{ext} \tag{2.12}$$

where:

$$\mathbf{M}_e^s = \int_{\Omega^e} \rho\mathbf{N}^{\mathrm{T}}\mathbf{N}\mathrm{d}\Omega \tag{2.13}$$

$$\mathbf{K}_e^s = \int_{\Omega^e} \mathbf{B}\cdot\mathbf{D}\mathbf{B}\mathrm{d}\Omega \tag{2.14}$$

$$\mathbf{f}_e^{ext} - \text{external force} = \int_{S_t} \mathbf{N}^{\mathrm{T}}\bar{\mathbf{t}}^{\mathrm{T}} dS + \int_V \mathbf{N}^{\mathrm{T}}\bar{\mathbf{b}}^{\mathrm{T}} dV \tag{2.15}$$

Assemble the matrixes of elements to form the global form:

$$\mathbf{M}^s\mathbf{u} + \mathbf{K}^s\mathbf{u} = \mathbf{f}^s \tag{2.16}$$

where:

$$\mathbf{M}^s = \sum \mathbf{M}_e^s \tag{2.17}$$

$$\mathbf{K}^s = \sum \mathbf{K}_e^s \tag{2.18}$$

$$\mathbf{f}^s = \sum \mathbf{f}_e^{ext} \tag{2.19}$$

The external forces in Equation (2.16) can be: (1) fluid pressure in fluid-structure interaction; (2) acoustic pressure in acoustic fluid-structure interaction; and (3) thermal force in thermal-structural analysis.

In the case of existing damping, Equation (2.16) becomes:

$$\mathbf{M}^s\mathbf{u} + \mathbf{C}^s\dot{\mathbf{u}} + \mathbf{K}^s\mathbf{u} = \mathbf{f}^s \tag{2.20}$$

where $\mathbf{C}^s$ is the damping matrix.

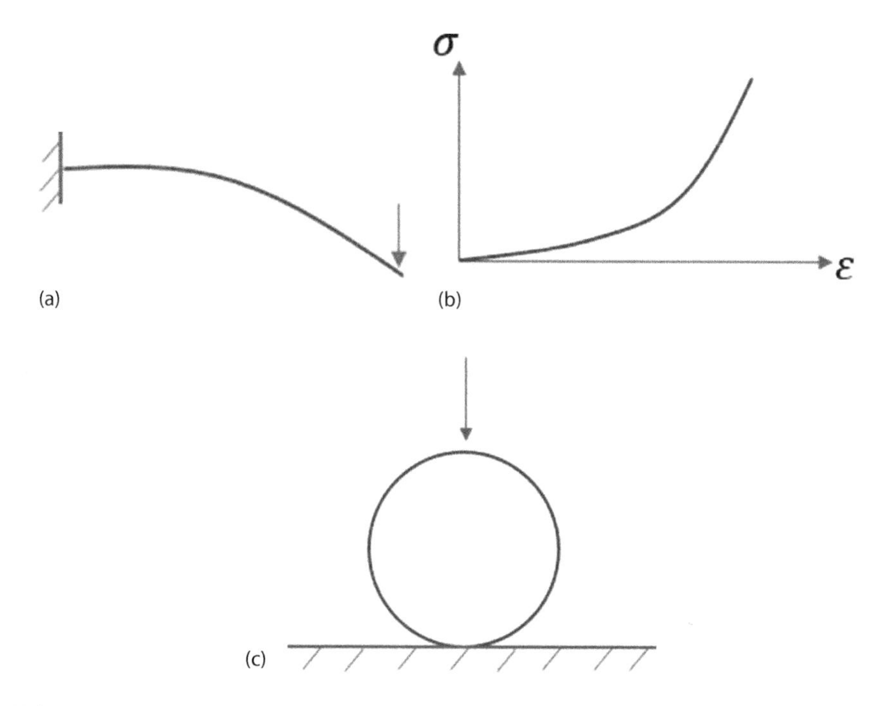

FIGURE 2.3 Various nonlinearities (a) large deformation; (b) nonlinear material; and (c) contact.

Although Equation (2.20) is derived based on assumptions of the linear elasticity with small strains, it works for the general nonlinear conditions [4]. In practice, Equation (2.20) can be nonlinear due to the following three factors:

1. *Large strain*: When the large strain occurs (Figure 2.3a), the last term in the Equation (2.3) cannot be negligible; this makes the internal force in Equation (2.8) very complicated.
2. *Nonlinear stress-strain relations*: Stress-strain relations in many engineering problems can be simplified as linear. However, some materials, such as hyperelastic materials (Figure 2.3b) and nonlinear elastoplastic materials, are strongly nonlinear. Reference [6] gives the details of various nonlinear material models.
3. *Contact*: The contact status of the contact surfaces between two bodies changes with loadings (Figure 2.3c). Thus, different constraint conditions added in Equation (2.20) cause Equation (2.20) to be nonlinear.

Nonlinear Equation (2.20) is always solved by the Newton-Raphson method (Figure 2.4) that makes the residual very small with successive corrections until the tolerance is reached.

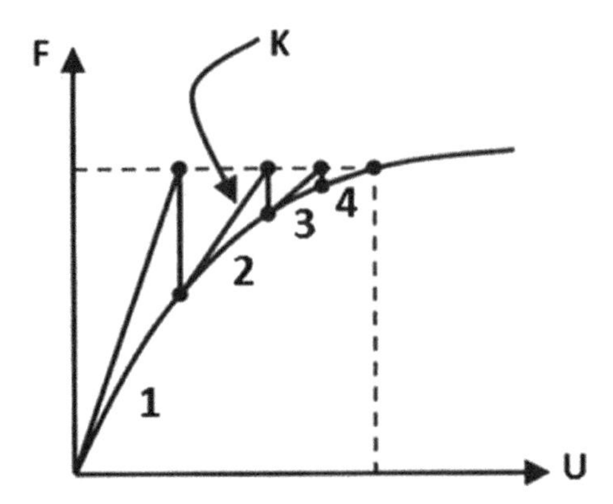

FIGURE 2.4 Schematic of Newton-Raphson method.

2.3 FINITE ELEMENT PROCEDURE OF STRUCTURAL ANALYSIS IN ANSYS

The general procedure to build a finite element model is listed in Figure 2.5. The following gives the specific procedure to build a finite element model in ANSYS for structural analysis:

1. *Build the model*: A structural model can be built in the pre-process of MAPDL and ANSYS Workbench. It also can be created in other computer aided design (CAD) software and imported into ANSYS.
2. *Set up the model environment*: Different element types are available in ANSYS, such as Plane 182/183 for two-dimensional models, SOLID185/186/187 for three-dimensional models, Shell 181/281 for shell models, and Beam 188/189 for beam models.
3. *Define the material properties*: The linear and nonlinear material properties can be defined by the MP or TB commands in ANSYS.
4. *Mesh the model*: After the element types and material properties are defined, the geometry obtained in step 1 can be meshed in MAPDL and the Workbench using the meshing tool. The ideal meshing has regular element shapes and fine meshing sizes applied for the area with high stress gradients.
5. *Define loadings and the boundary conditions*: The force loadings and displacement boundary conditions are specified in ANSYS using F, D, and relevant commands.
6. *Solve the equation*: Sparse solver is widely used to solve the structural analysis. The linear problem can be solved in one sub-step, but the nonlinear problem may need many sub-steps before completion.
7. *Post-process the analysis*: After the solution, the deformation and stress distribution can be plotted using PLNSOL/PRNSOL/PLESOL/PRESOL commands in a POST1 post-processor. A POST26 post-processor shows the time history of the results of nodes and elements.

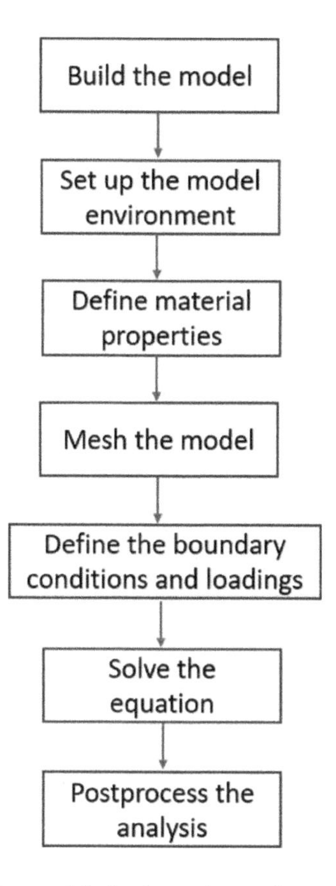

FIGURE 2.5 Flow chart of general finite element procedure.

2.4 DEFORMATION OF INTERVERTEBRAL DISC UNDER COMPRESSION

Clinical studies indicate that about 31 million Americans suffer back pain in their lifetime [7]. The mechanics of load transfer to the intervertebral disc is crucial for understanding the patterns and mechanisms of back pain. Therefore, it is necessary to build a finite element model of the intervertebral disc to study its stress state.

2.4.1 Finite Element Model

A finite element model of the intervertebral disc (IVD), which is composed of the endplates, nucleus, and annulus, was created. The IVD was assumed symmetrical. Thus, half an IVD was modeled (Figure 2.6b), and its dimensions are given in Figure 2.6c. The model, including 6,614 elements and 7,870 nodes, was meshed with SOLID185 in ANSYS.

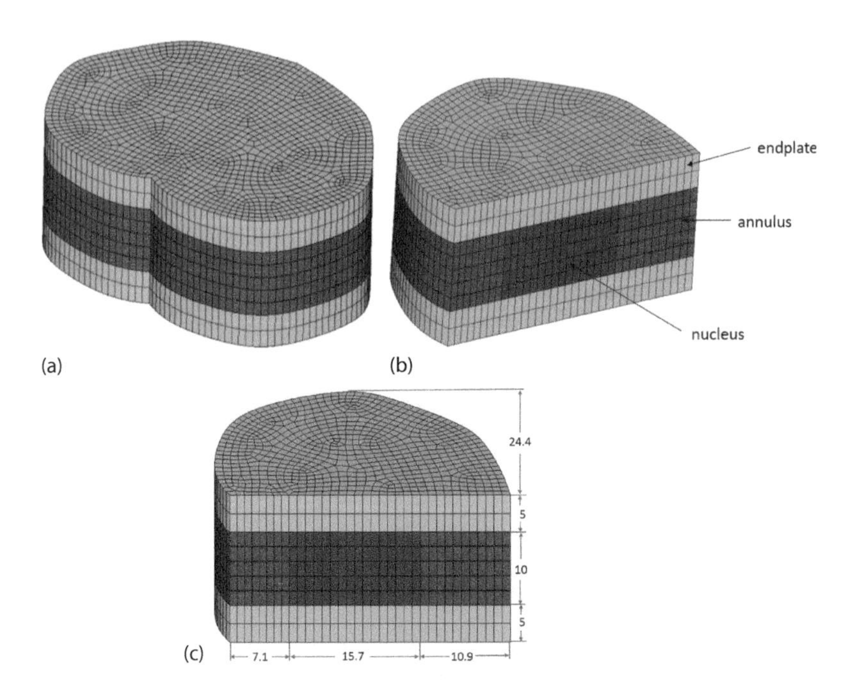

FIGURE 2.6 Finite element model of IVD (a) full model of IVD; (b) half model of IVD; and (c) dimensions of IVD (all dimensions in mm).

2.4.2 Material Properties

The materials of the IVD were assumed linear elastic. Their material parameters are listed in Table 2.1 [8].

2.4.3 Boundary Conditions and Loadings

The bottom of the IVD was fixed and the symmetrical condition was applied (Figure 2.7a). The top surface of the endplate was loaded with pressure, which was ramp-loaded to 0.5 MPa in the first step, and then unloaded to zero in the second step (Figure 2.7b).

TABLE 2.1
Material Parameters of the IVD

	Young's Modulus (MPa)	Poisson's Ratio
Endplate	3,500	0.3
Nucleus	0.15	0.17
Annulus	1.5	0.17

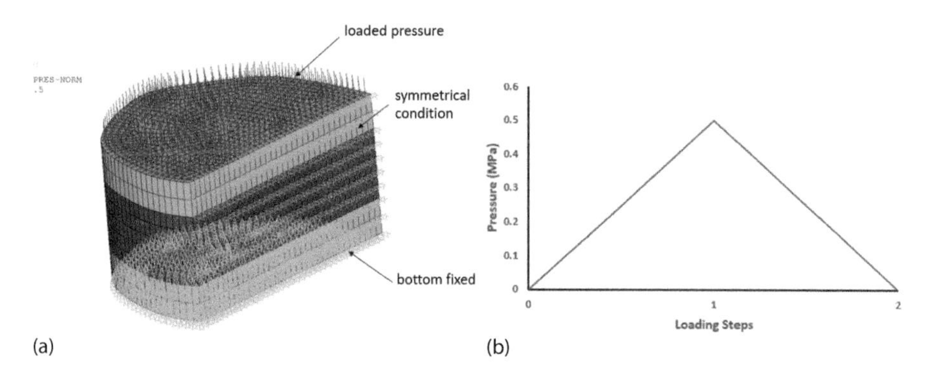

FIGURE 2.7 Loadings and boundary conditions (a) loadings and boundary conditions and (b) time history of pressure loading.

2.4.4 Solution Setting

The pressure peak is 0.5 MPa, which is relatively high compared to the Young's modulus of nucleus and annulus. Thus, large deflection effects should be turned on by the command NLGEOM, ON [9].

2.4.5 Results

Figure 2.8 plots the deformation of the IVD in the first and second steps. At the end of the first step, with the loaded pressure, the IVD was compressed in the vertical direction, and the annulus extended in the axial direction, which formed a bulging disc. In the second step, after the pressure was gone, the IVD recovered to the initial shape, and the bulging disc disappeared.

The stresses and strains of the IVD in the first and second steps are illustrated in Figures 2.9 and 2.10. The maximum strain 0.567 indicates that large deflection effects are necessary in the solution setting.

Because the bone is about 2,000 times stiffer than the nucleus and annulus, the bone can be regarded as rigid, which causes the top surface of the annulus and the nucleus connected to the bone to have a uniform deformation in the vertical direction. As a result, the annulus and the nucleus have relatively constant strains except at the edges. Because the Young's modulus of the nucleus is given as one-tenth of the annulus (Table 2.1), the stresses are mainly shown in the annulus (Figure 2.10). With loading gone in the second step, the strains and stresses in the second step were close to zero.

Figure 2.11 presents the vertical displacement of the IVD with time, which clearly shows that it increases in the first step to peak value 3.5 mm, and then goes back to the initial position in the second unloading stage. The loading/unloading curve is not linear because of the large deformation of the annulus and nucleus.

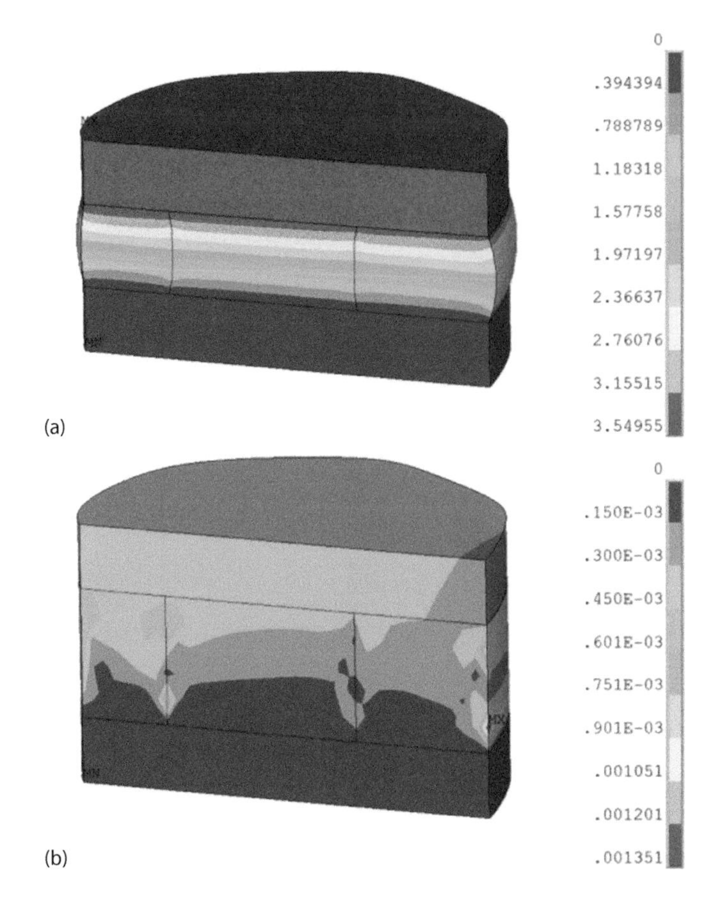

FIGURE 2.8 Displacement of IVD (a) displacement of IVD at the end of the first step (mm) and (b) displacement of IVD at the end of the last step (mm).

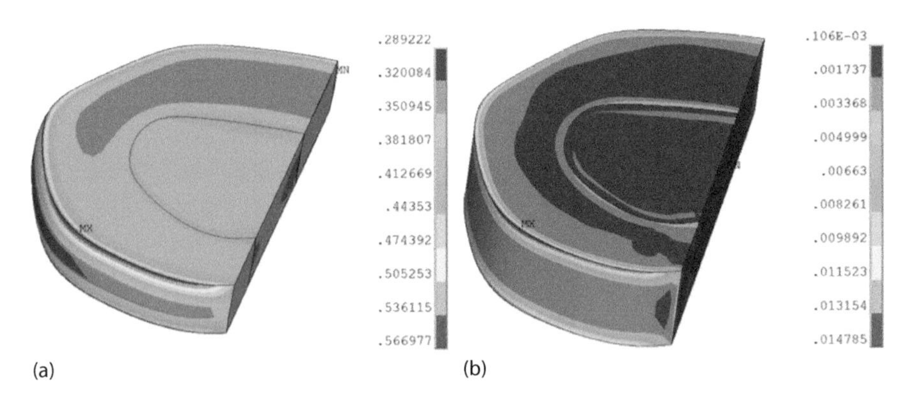

FIGURE 2.9 vM strains of IVD (a) vM strains of IVD at the end of the first step and (b) vM strains of IVD at the end of the last step.

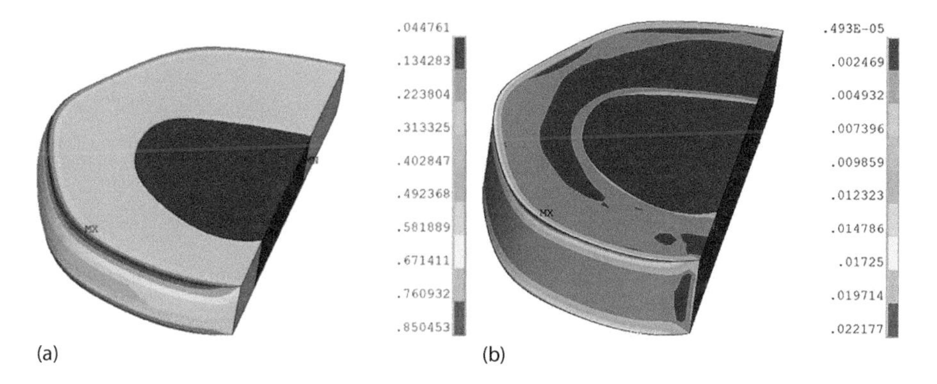

FIGURE 2.10 vM stresses of IVD (a) vM stresses of IVD at the end of the first step (MPa) and (b) vM stresses of IVD at the end of the last step (MPa).

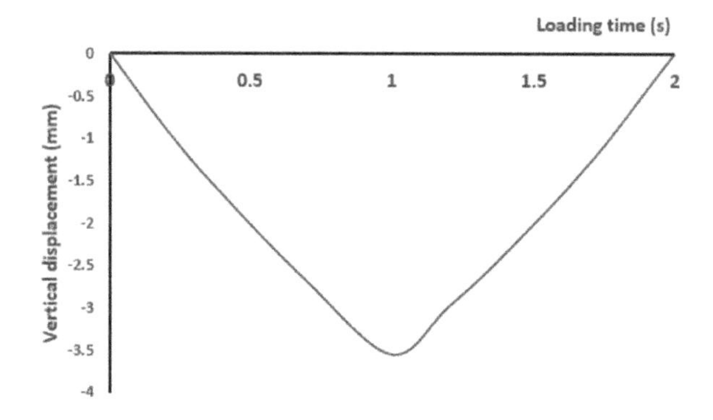

FIGURE 2.11 Vertical displacement versus loading time.

2.4.6 Discussion

A three-dimensional finite element model of the intervertebral disc was created. Under compression, the bulging disc was formed, which matched the clinical observation.

The materials of the nucleus and annulus were assumed linear and elastic. That is why the IVD recovers fully after the loading is removed. Obviously, the linear elastic material for the nucleus and annulus was simplified, because the nucleus and annulus contain about 70% and 30% of water, respectively. Therefore, it is more appropriate to model them as porous media. One example in [10] modeled the nucleus and annulus with coupled pore-pressure thermal elements to simulate the creep of IVD in ANSYS.

2.4.7 Summary

The deformation of the intervertebral disc was simulated in ANSYS. The bulging disc appeared when the intervertebral disc was under compression and disappeared when the loading was gone.

REFERENCES

1. Andriacchi, T.P., Mundermann, A., Smith, R.L., Alexander, E.J., Dyrby, C.O., and Koo, S., "A framework for the *in vivo* pathomechanics of osteoarthritis at the knee," *Annals of Biomedical Engineering*, Vol. 32, 2004, pp. 447–457.
2. Sarda, V., Handa, A.C., and Arora, K.K., *Chemistry Part I*, New Saraswati House Pvt. Ltd., New Delhi, 2016.
3. Belytschko, T., Liu, W.K., Moran, B., and Elkhodary, K., *Nonlinear Finite Elements for Continua and Structures*, Wiley, Hoboken, NJ, 2000.
4. Zhang, Q., and Cen, S., *Multiphysics Modeling: Numerical Methods and Engineering Applications*, Academic Press, Cambridge, MA, 2016.
5. Dill, E.H., *The Finite Element Method for Mechanics of Solids with ANSYS Applications*, CRC Press, Boca Raton, FL, 2012.
6. Yang, Z., *Material Modeling in Finite Element Analysis*, CRC Press, Boca Raton, FL, 2019.
7. Jensen, M.C., Brant-Zawadzki, M.N., Obuchowski, N., Modic, M.T., Malkasian, D., and Ross, J.S., "Magnetic resonance imaging of the lumbar spine in people without back pain," *New England Journal of Medicine*, Vol. 331, 1994, pp. 69–116.
8. Schroeder, Y., Wilson, W., Huyghe, J.M., and Baaijens, F.P.T., "Osmoviscoelastic finite element model of the intervertebral disc," *European Spine Journal*, Vol. 15 (Suppl. 3), 2006, pp. S361–S371.
9. ANSYS Help Documentation in the help page of Product ANSYS190, 2018.
10. Yang, Z., *Finite Element Analysis for Biomedical Engineering Applications*, CRC Press, Boca Raton, FL, 2019.

3 Fluid Analysis

Fluid flow, such as blood in the vessel, air in the lungs, and urine through the ureter, exists in the human body. Thus, computational fluid dynamics (CFD) has been applied in biomedical studies.

Unlike the solid phase discussed in Chapter 2, fluid, the subject of Chapter 3, continuously changes shape under external forces. The governing equations of fluid flow and modeling procedure in ANSYS Fluent, as well as the application for the modeling of blood flow through a stenotic artery, are presented in Chapter 3.

3.1 NATURE OF FLUIDS

In contrast to solids, fluids lack the ability to resist deformation. Thus, a fluid moves under the action of the force. Its shape changes continuously in response to external forces (Figure 3.1) [1]. In addition, a fluid is prone to stick to itself. When one element of a fluid moves, it tends to carry others with it. Therefore, no abrupt discontinuity exists in the velocity of fluids. The velocity continuously changes within a transition region. Furthermore, fluids do not slip with respect to solids, which makes the velocity of the fluid at a solid interface the same as the velocity of the solid. Consequently, a boundary layer forms near a solid interface (Figure 3.2).

Fluids have various compressible behaviors. It is well known that gases can be more easily compressed than liquids. In computational fluid dynamics, water is always regarded as incompressible.

3.2 GOVERNING EQUATIONS OF FLUIDS AND THEIR NUMERICAL SIMULATION

3.2.1 Eulerian Description

Because the shape of the fluid changes continuously, the Lagrangian description is no longer applicable for the fluid. Therefore, another approach—the Eulerian description—is adopted, in which the fluid flow properties are expressed as fields

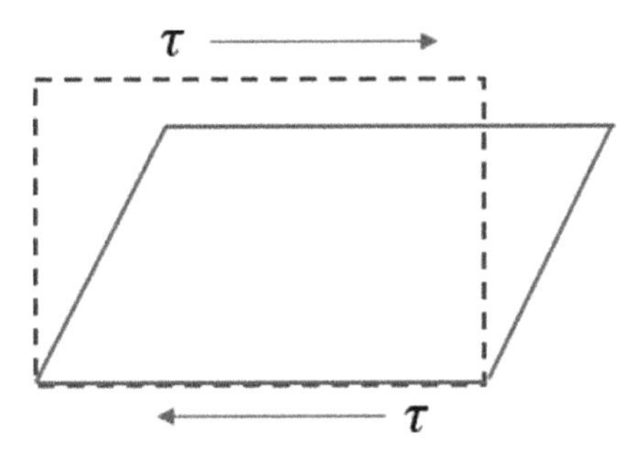

FIGURE 3.1 Fluid loaded with shear force.

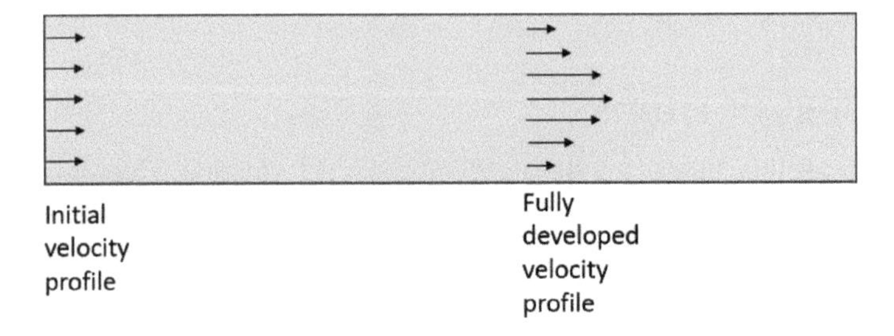

FIGURE 3.2 Boundary layer of fluid.

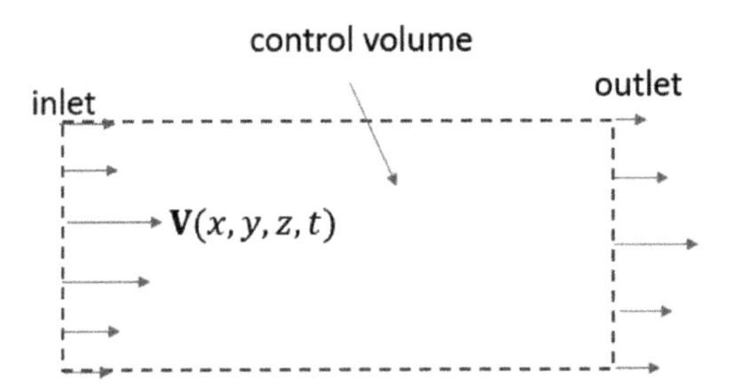

FIGURE 3.3 Eulerian description.

once a control volume is defined (Figure 3.3). Unlike the Lagrangian description, the Eulerian description does not identify individual particles. Instead, within a control volume, pressure, velocity, acceleration, and other flow properties are defined as fields [2]:

In space (x, y, and z) and time t,

Pressure field: $p = p(x, y, z, t)$

Velocity field: $\mathbf{v} = \mathbf{v}(x, y, z, t)$

Acceleration field: $\mathbf{a} = \mathbf{a}(x, y, z, t)$

3.2.2 Governing Equations

1. *Conservation of mass*: The partial equation of the conservation law can be written in the following form [3]:

$$\frac{\partial \rho}{\partial t} + \nabla \cdot \rho \mathbf{v} = 0 \tag{3.1}$$

2. *Conservation of momentum*: The differential form of the conservation of an inviscid fluid is given as [3]:

$$\frac{\partial}{\partial t}(\rho \mathbf{v}) + \nabla \cdot (\rho \mathbf{v}\mathbf{v}) + \nabla p - \rho \mathbf{b} = 0 \tag{3.2}$$

For the incompressible fluids, Equation (3.1) is a function of velocity and has no pressure term there. Equation (3.2) contains both velocity and pressure terms. The weak coupling of the velocity and pressure fields leads to one of the most widely used algorithms for the incompressible flow—Semi-Implicit Method for Pressure Linked Equations (SIMPLE) algorithm [3]—to solve Equations (3.1) and (3.2). In the SIMPLE algorithm, the velocity components are first computed from the momentum equations using an estimated pressure field. Then, the pressure and velocities are adjusted to satisfy the continuity equation. The convergence is reached after many iterations of the procedure (Figure 3.4).

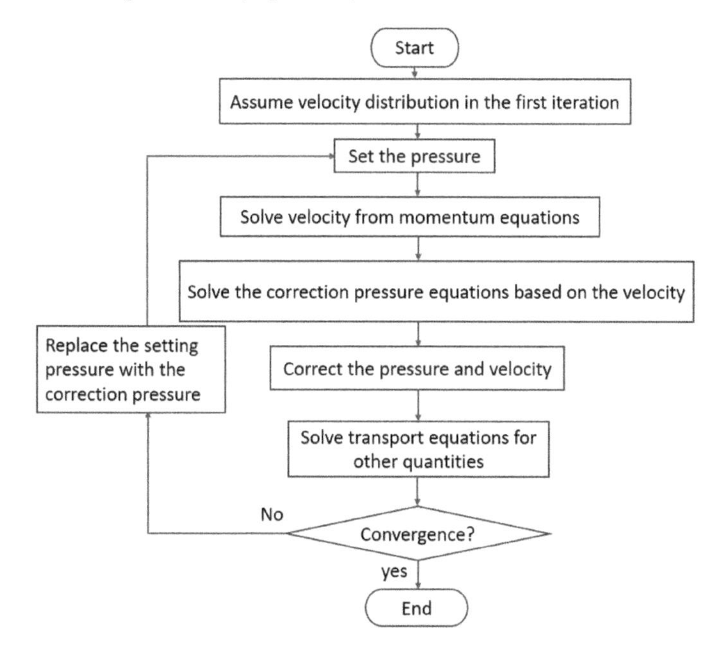

FIGURE 3.4 Flow chart of SIMPLE algorithm.

3.3 MODELING PROCEDURE IN ANSYS FLUENT

Equations (3.1) and (3.2) can be solved by the finite difference method, finite element method, and finite volume method. ANSYS Fluent adopts the finite volume method. The general procedure to build one CFD model in ANSYS Fluent is listed as follows:

1. *Build the model*: A model can be built in the SpaceClaim. It also can be created in other computer-aided design (CAD) software and imported into ANSYS workbench.
2. *Mesh the model*: The ideal meshing has regular element shapes. As the boundary layer exists in the model, the meshing close to the wall should be very fine.
3. *Physical model*: The fluid flow is classified into laminar and turbulent flows. They can be identified by Reynolds numbers and specified in ANSYS Fluent.
4. *Define the material properties*: The fluid divided into air and liquid, along with the density and dynamic viscosity of the fluid, should be defined.
5. *Define the boundary conditions*: The pressure and velocity are specified in the inlet and outlet of the control volume.
6. *Run calculation*: In the run calculation, the time step size and number of time steps, as well as max iteration, should be assigned.
7. *Post-process the analysis*: After solution, the pressure and velocity contours can be plotted in the post-process.

3.4 STUDY OF BLOOD FLOW THROUGH A STENOTIC ARTERY BY CFD

The function of blood vessels is to carry blood throughout the body. The blood vessel consists of arteries, which can experience atherosclerosis caused by the formation of fat, cells, and other substances. The hardening causes the blood vessel to narrow, making it more difficult for the blood to flow. Under such flowing conditions, the artery may experience high shear stresses and blood recirculation [4]. This study tried to simulate blood flow through a stenotic artery in ANSYS Fluent.

3.4.1 Finite Element Model

A 180×6 mm rectangle with narrowing 80% in the middle was used to represent an axisymmetrical stenotic artery (Figure 3.5). The blood flow was pushed by a pulsatile pressure drop between the inlet and outlet, which is expressed as [5]:

$$\frac{\Delta P}{\rho v^2} = 0.225 + 1.5 \sin\left(2\pi ft\right) \tag{3.3}$$

where:

$f = 1.25$ Hz;

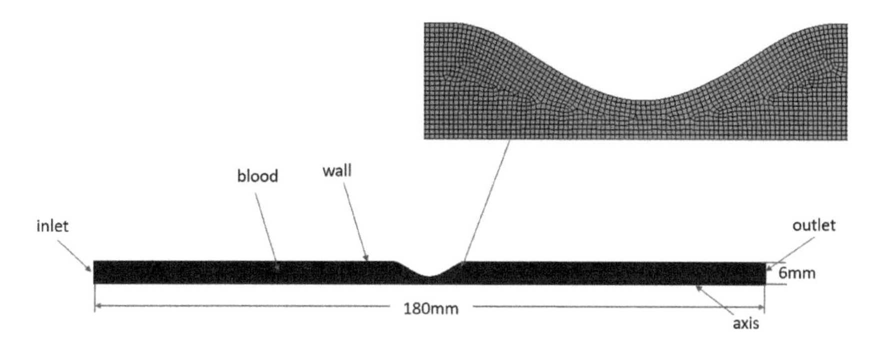

FIGURE 3.5 Model of a stenotic artery.

$\rho = 1{,}050 \text{ kg/m}^3$; and
$v = 0.59 \text{ m/s}$.

Thus, the pressure defined as a function of time was implemented in the following user-defined function (udf) file:

```
#include "udf.h"
DEFINE_PROFILE(unsteady_pressure, thread, position)
{
real t=CURRENT_TIME;
face_t f;

begin_f_loop(f,thread)
{
F_PROFILE(f,thread,position) = (1050*0.59*0.59*(0.225+1.5*sin(
2*3.1416*1.25*t)));
}
end_f_loop(f,thread)
}
```

The time-average Reynolds number is Rem = 410, and the Womersley number is $\alpha = 13.1$ [6]. Thus, the flow was regarded as laminar.

The CFD analysis was performed in ANSYS Fluent through the following steps:

1. build geometry of blood vessel, and mesh it;
2. specify model as two-dimensional axisymmetrical;
3. define simulation as transient;
4. specify the flow as laminar;
5. define density 1,050 kg/m^3 and dynamic viscosity 0.0035 Pa.s in the material properties;
6. specify the pressure at the inlet using the above udf file and outlet as zero;
7. assign time step size and total number steps as 0.1 seconds and 20, respectively; and
8. run the transient flow simulation.

3.4.2 Results

Figure 3.6 illustrates the residuals with iterations, which show that the convergence is reached in continuity, x-velocity, and y-velocity. The whole flow field of velocity, static pressure, and total pressure at time 2 seconds are presented in Figures 3.7 through 3.9. For comparison, the corresponding results of the normal vessel are given in Figures 3.10 through 3.12. The results clearly show that the pressure and the velocity change dramatically at the narrowing area. The maximum velocity is 1.05 m/s at the stenotic artery, which is much higher than 0.558 m/s at the normal artery. Similarly, the peak value of total pressure at the stenotic artery is 445 Pa, which is much higher than 163 Pa at the normal artery.

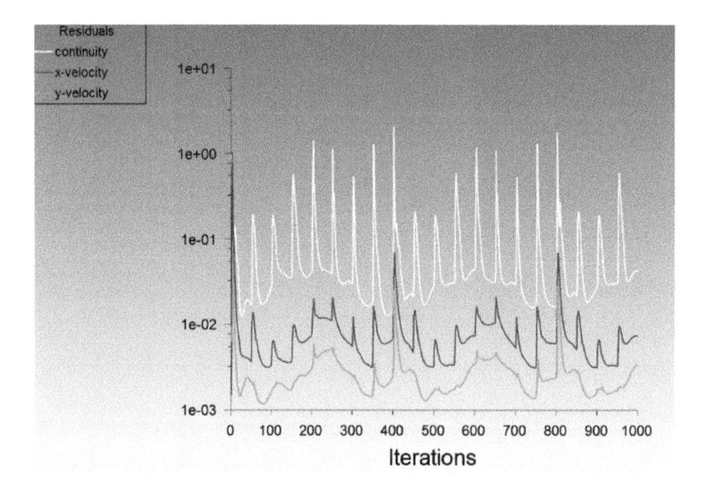

FIGURE 3.6 Residuals with iterations.

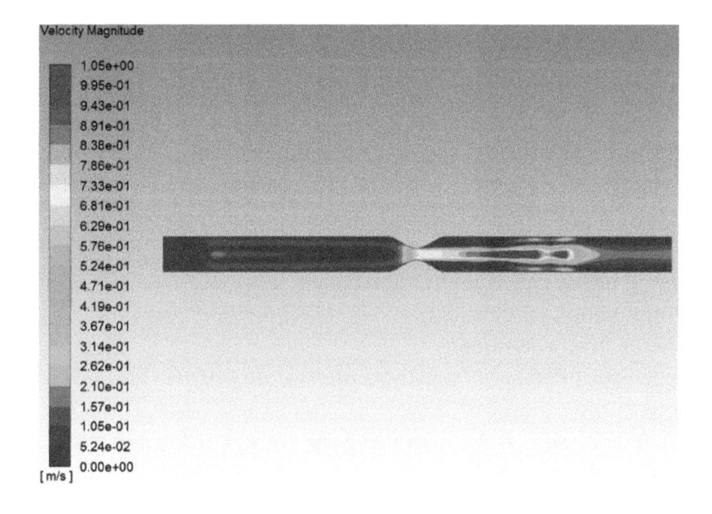

FIGURE 3.7 Contour of final flow velocity of the stenotic artery.

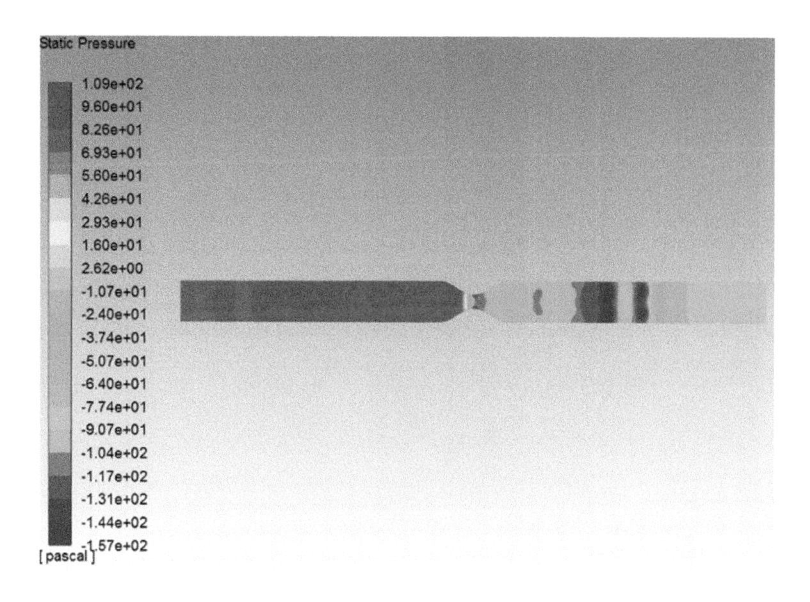

FIGURE 3.8 Contour of final static pressure of the stenotic artery.

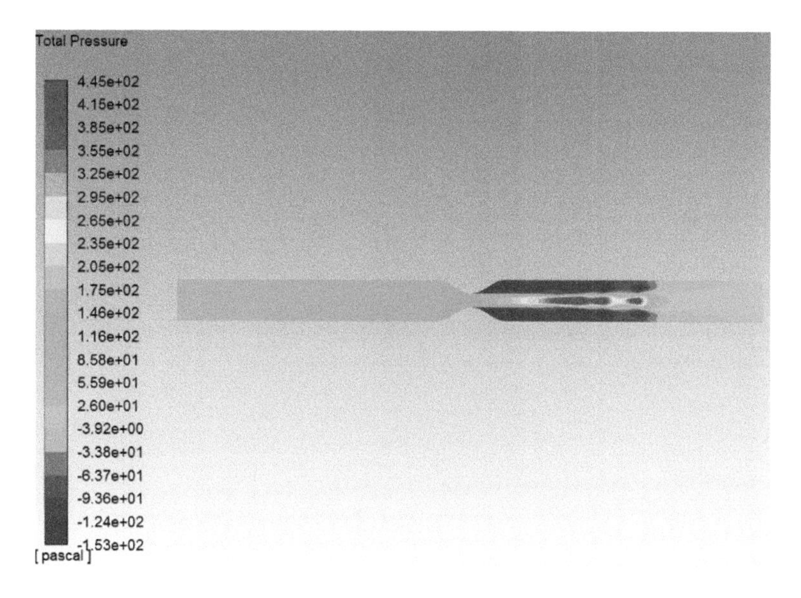

FIGURE 3.9 Contour of final total pressure of the stenotic artery.

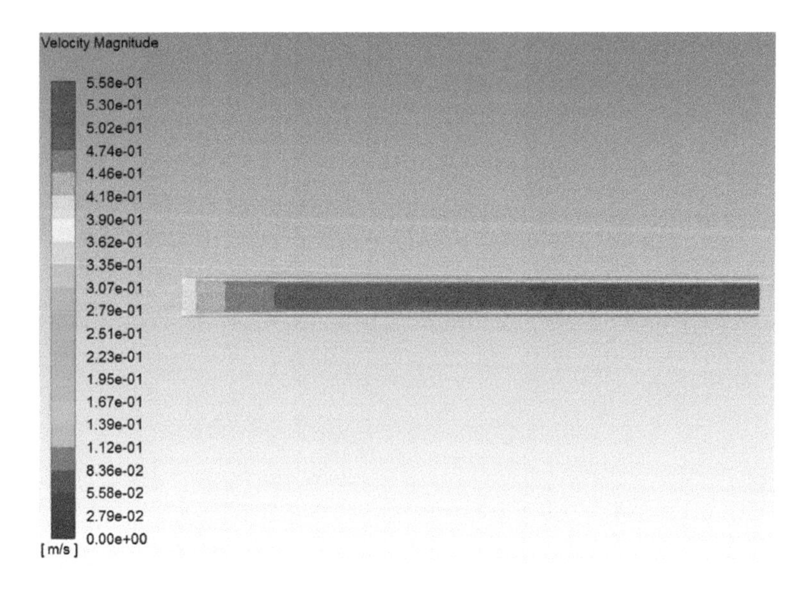

FIGURE 3.10 Contour of final flow velocity of the normal artery.

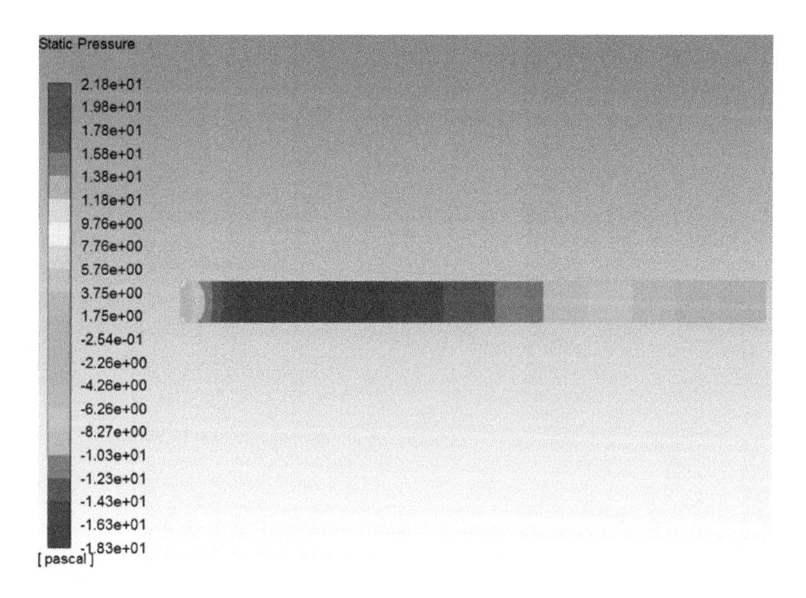

FIGURE 3.11 Contour of final static pressure of the normal artery.

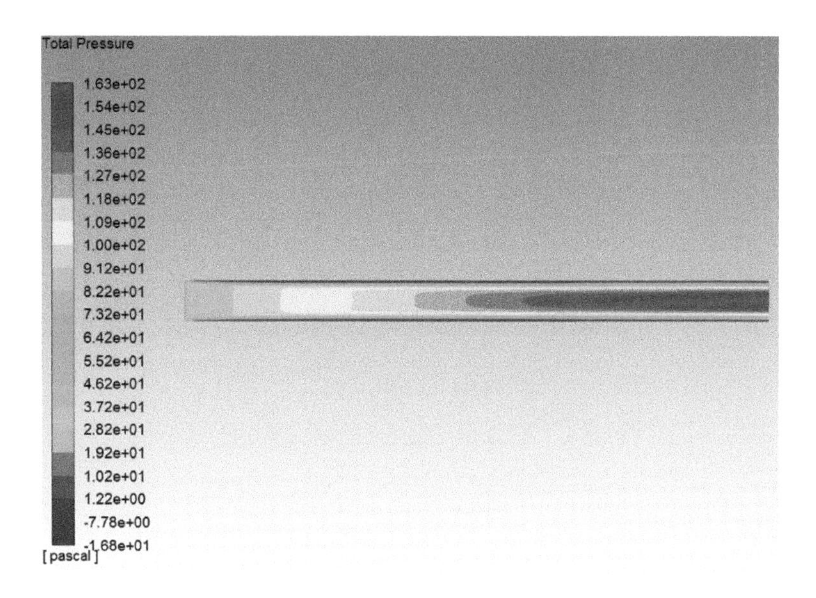

FIGURE 3.12 Contour of final total pressure of the normal artery.

3.4.3 Summary

Blood flow through a stenotic artery was simulated in ANSYS Fluent, and the convergence was reached in continuity, x-velocity, and y-velocity. The computational results clearly show that the pressure and the velocity change dramatically at the narrowing area.

REFERENCES

1. Smits, A.J., *A Physical Introduction to Fluid Mechanics*, Wiley, Hoboken, NJ, 1999.
2. https://www.me.psu.edu/cimbala/Learning/Fluid/Introductory/descriptions_of_fluid_flows.htm
3. Moukalled, F., Mangani, L., and Darwish, M., *The Finite Volume Method in Computational Fluid Dynamics*, Springer, New York, 2015.
4. Tang, D., Yang, C., Zheng, J., and Vito, R.P., "Stress/strain analysis of arteries with stenotic plaques and lipid cores," In *Proceedings of the Fourth World Congress of Biomechanics*, Calgary, August 4–9, 2002.
5. Khalili, F., *Fluid Dynamics Modeling and Sound Analysis of a Bileaflet Mechanical Heart Valve*, PhD dissertation, University of Central Florida, 2018.
6. Scotti, C.M., Shkolnik, A.D., Muluk, S.C., and Finol, E.A., "Fluid-structure interaction in abdominal aortic aneurysms: Effects of asymmetry and wall thickness," *Bio Medical Engineering OnLine*, Vol. 4, 2005, p. 64.

4 Acoustic Analysis

The ear diseases are often connected with the sound wave in the ear. For example, big blasts on the battlefield cause the injuries of the tympanic membrane [1,2]. Therefore, the acoustic analysis has been applied to biomedical research.

Sound is a wave characterized by the wave equations. Chapter 4 discusses sound, including its governing equation and finite element implementation, and gives an acoustic analysis of a body under a blast in an open area.

4.1 SOUND WAVES

Sound waves propagate in a fluid with a form of compressional oscillatory disturbances. Sound waves are longitudinal waves, in which the particles move back and forth along the direction of propagation. The sound pressure is the difference between the instant value of the total pressure and the static pressure. In most cases, the sound pressure compared with the static pressure is extremely small. For example, the ratio of a sound pressure of 120 dB to the static pressure is about 2e-4, although 120 dB is close to the threshold of pain.

Sound waves reveal some characteristics of waves, including interference, reflection, and diffraction (Figure 4.1) [3].

4.2 GOVERNING EQUATION AND FINITE ELEMENT IMPLEMENTATION

The acoustic fluid is assumed to be:

1. compressible;
2. inviscid or nonviscous;
3. without mean flow of the fluid; and
4. with uniform mean density and pressure throughout the fluid.

Then, the acoustic fluid with the above assumption is governed by the continuity equation:

$$\frac{\partial \rho}{\partial t} + \rho_0 \frac{\partial v_i}{\partial x_i} = 0 \tag{4.1}$$

and momentum equation:

$$\rho_0 \frac{\partial v_i}{\partial t} = -\frac{\partial p}{\partial x_i} \tag{4.2}$$

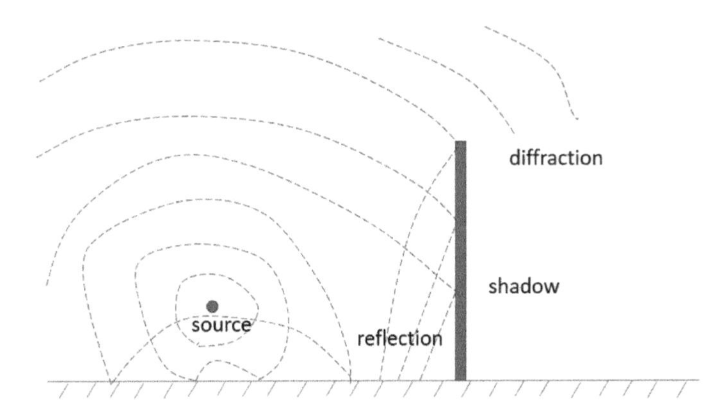

FIGURE 4.1 Various wave phenomena. (From www.pearl-hifi.com/06_Lit_Archive/14_Books_Tech_Papers/Introduction_to_Acoustics.pdf.)

The state equation is expressed as:

$$p = c^2 \rho \tag{4.3}$$

where c is the speed of sound in a fluid medium.

Taking derivative of t and x_i of Equations (4.1) and (4.2), respectively, and then combining both equations results in the following:

$$\frac{\partial^2 \rho}{\partial t^2} - \frac{\partial^2 p}{\partial x_i^2} = 0 \tag{4.4}$$

Substituting Equation (4.3) into the above equation to remove term ρ[4] leads to the following:

$$\frac{1}{c^2}\frac{\partial^2 p}{\partial t^2} - \frac{\partial^2 p}{\partial x_i^2} = 0 \tag{4.5}$$

Multiplying Equation (4.5) by a virtual change in pressure, and integrating it over the volume of domain obtains the following equation:

$$\int_{\Omega_f} \frac{1}{c^2}\delta p \frac{\partial^2 p}{\partial t^2} \mathrm{d}\Omega + \int_{\Omega_f} \frac{\partial(\delta p)}{\partial x_i}\frac{\partial p}{\partial x_i} \mathrm{d}\Omega = 0 \tag{4.6}$$

where:

Ω_f = volume of domain and
δp = a virtual change in pressure.

When the dissipation occurs at the boundary surface Γ_0, a dissipation term, is added in the left side of the above equation:

$$\int_{\Omega_f} \frac{1}{c^2} \delta p \frac{\partial^2 p}{\partial t^2} \mathrm{d}\Omega + \int_{\Omega_f} \frac{\partial(\delta p)}{\partial x_i} \frac{\partial p}{\partial x_i} \mathrm{d}\Omega + \int_{\Gamma_0} \delta p \left[\frac{r}{\rho_0 c} \right] \frac{1}{c} \frac{\partial p}{\partial t} \mathrm{d}\Gamma = 0 \tag{4.7}$$

The shape functions for the acoustic pressure is expressed by:

$$p = \mathbf{N}_p^{\mathrm{T}} \mathbf{p}_e \tag{4.8}$$

where:

$\mathbf{N}_p$ = element shape function of pressure and

$\mathbf{p}_e$ = element nodal pressure vector.

Therefore,

$$\frac{\partial p}{\partial t} = \mathbf{N}_p^{\mathrm{T}} \dot{\mathbf{p}}_e = \dot{\mathbf{p}}_e{}^{\mathrm{T}} \mathbf{N}_p \tag{4.9}$$

$$\frac{\partial^2 p}{\partial t^2} = \mathbf{N}_p^{\mathrm{T}} \ddot{\mathbf{p}}_e = \ddot{\mathbf{p}}_e{}^{\mathrm{T}} \mathbf{N}_p \tag{4.10}$$

$$\frac{\partial p}{\partial x_i} = \frac{\partial \mathbf{N}_p^{\mathrm{T}} \mathbf{p}_e}{\partial x_i} = \frac{\partial \mathbf{N}_p^{\mathrm{T}}}{\partial x_i} \mathbf{p}_e = \mathbf{B}_p \mathbf{p}_e \tag{4.11}$$

where $\mathbf{B}_{ji} = \frac{\partial \mathbf{N}_j}{\partial x_i}$, j is the node index of one element.

Substituting Equations (4.9)–(4.11) into the weak form Equation (4.7) yields the matrix form of the acoustic equation:

$$\mathbf{M}_e^p \ddot{\mathbf{p}}_e + \mathbf{C}_e^p \dot{\mathbf{p}}_e + \mathbf{K}_e^p \mathbf{p}_e = 0 \tag{4.12}$$

where:

$\mathbf{M}_e^p$ = acoustic mass matrix,

$$= \frac{1}{c^2} \int_{\Omega_e} \mathbf{N}_p \mathbf{N}_p^{\mathrm{T}} \mathrm{d}\Omega \tag{4.13}$$

$\mathbf{C}_e^p$ = acoustic damping matrix,

$$= \frac{r}{\rho_0 c^2} \int_{\Gamma_0} \mathbf{N}_p \mathbf{N}_p^{\mathrm{T}} \mathrm{d}\Gamma \tag{4.14}$$

$\mathbf{K}_e^p$ = acoustic stiffness matrix,

$$= \int_{\Omega_f} \mathbf{B}_p^{\mathrm{T}} \mathbf{B}_p \mathrm{d}\Omega \tag{4.15}$$

Assembling element Equation (4.12) into the global matrix as [5]:

$$\mathbf{M}^p\ddot{\mathbf{p}} + \mathbf{C}^p\dot{\mathbf{p}} + \mathbf{K}^p\mathbf{p} = 0 \tag{4.16}$$

where:

$$\mathbf{M}^p = \sum \mathbf{M}_e^p \tag{4.17}$$

$$\mathbf{C}^p = \sum \mathbf{C}_e^p \tag{4.18}$$

$$\mathbf{K}^p = \sum \mathbf{K}_e^p \tag{4.19}$$

Equation (4.16) is linear and can be solved by the sparse solver. This equation was implemented in ANSYS as acoustic elements, including two-dimensional axisymmetrical acoustic elements Fluid 29 and three-dimensional acoustic elements Fluid30/220/221.

4.3 FINITE ELEMENT PROCEDURE IN ANSYS

The following steps outline the general procedure to build an acoustic finite element model [6]:

1. *Build the model*: An acoustic model consists of a fluid domain and the truncation of the infinite domain if the infinite domain exists. The model can be built in the ANSYS Workbench or by using other CAD software.
2. *Set up the model environment*: Two-dimensional axisymmetrical acoustic elements Fluid29 and three-dimensional acoustic elements Fluid30/220/221 are available in ANSYS to build the acoustic model.
3. *Define the material properties*: The acoustic material properties, such as density and sonic velocity, can be defined by MP or TB commands in ANSYS.
4. *Mesh the model*: In addition to the regular meshing requirement, ANSYS acoustic requires at least ten elements per wavelength for low-order elements or five elements per wavelength for high-order elements [6].
5. *Define the loadings and boundary conditions*: The acoustic loadings and boundary conditions are specified in ANSYS using SF, D, and BF commands.
6. *Solve the equation*: Sparse solver is widely used to solve the acoustic analysis, as acoustic Equation (4.16) is linear.
7. *Post-process the analysis*: After the solution, the acoustic quantity can be obtained using PRAS, PLAS commands in post-processing. The acoustic results are also plotted in both POST1 and POST26 of ANSYS.

4.4 ACOUSTIC ANALYSIS OF A BODY UNDER A BLAST IN AN OPEN AREA

This study simulated a body under a blast in an open area, which presents the general procedure to build an acoustic finite element model in ANSYS190.

4.4.1 Finite Element Model

The open area contained an acoustic source and a body. The distance between the acoustic source and the body was assumed to be 10 m. The acoustic source was modeled as a mass source, and the body was simplified as a cylinder with a radius of 0.5 m.

A 20 × 20 × 0.1 m block was created to simulate the open area, which was meshed by FLUID220. Because the harmonic analysis was conducted from 10 to 500 Hz, the maximum mesh size could be calculated by [6]:

$$\text{esize}_{\max} = \frac{\lambda}{6} = \frac{c}{6f} = 0.11\text{ m}. \tag{4.20}$$

Thus, mesh size 0.1 m was selected in this study.

Moreover, five perfectly matched layer (PML) elements were assigned with keyopt(4) = 1 to represent the infinite boundary (Figure 4.2) [6].

4.4.2 Material Properties

The density of the air and the speed of sound in the air were specified as 1.03 kg/m^3 and 340 m/s, respectively.

4.4.3 Loadings and Boundary Conditions

The five layers of PML elements presented the infinite boundary, in which the acoustic pressures were given as zero at the surface (Figure 4.3).

The mass source was defined by BF command:

```
NSEL, S, LOC, X, -4
NSEL, R, LOC, Y, -4
BF, ALL, MASS, 0.01
```

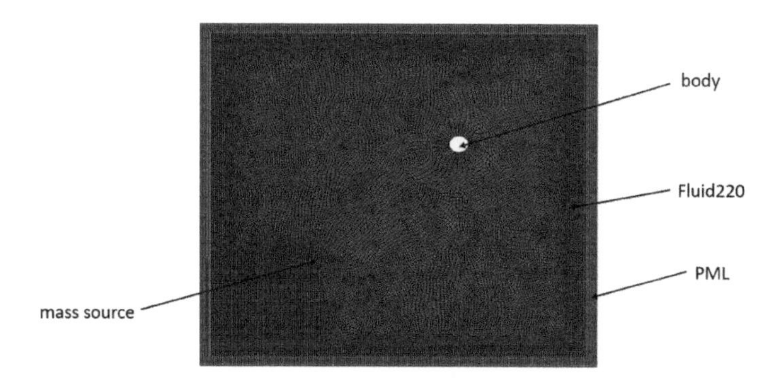

FIGURE 4.2 Acoustic model of a body under a blast in an open area.

FIGURE 4.3 PML boundary conditions.

4.4.4 Solution Setting

A harmonic analysis was conducted with the frequencies from 10 to 500 Hz.

4.4.5 Results

Figure 4.4 plots the acoustic pressures at different frequencies. At the low frequencies, such as 10 Hz, the body has little influence on the acoustic wave. With the increase of the frequencies, however, the interaction between the incident wave and reflected wave from the body becomes obvious.

The acoustic pressures at points A and B (Figure 4.5a) are presented in Figure 4.5b, which indicates that with the increase of frequencies, the acoustic pressures of A and B increase as well. However, the acoustic pressure of A is bigger than that of B, and their difference increases with the frequencies.

4.4.6 Discussion

The harmonic analysis of a body in the open area was completed in ANSYS190. The acoustic pressure contour at the high frequencies indicates the interaction between the incident wave and reflected wave.

This acoustic model is relatively simple. However, it incorporates the features of the acoustic models, such as PML elements for the infinite boundary and mesh size determined from the wavelength.

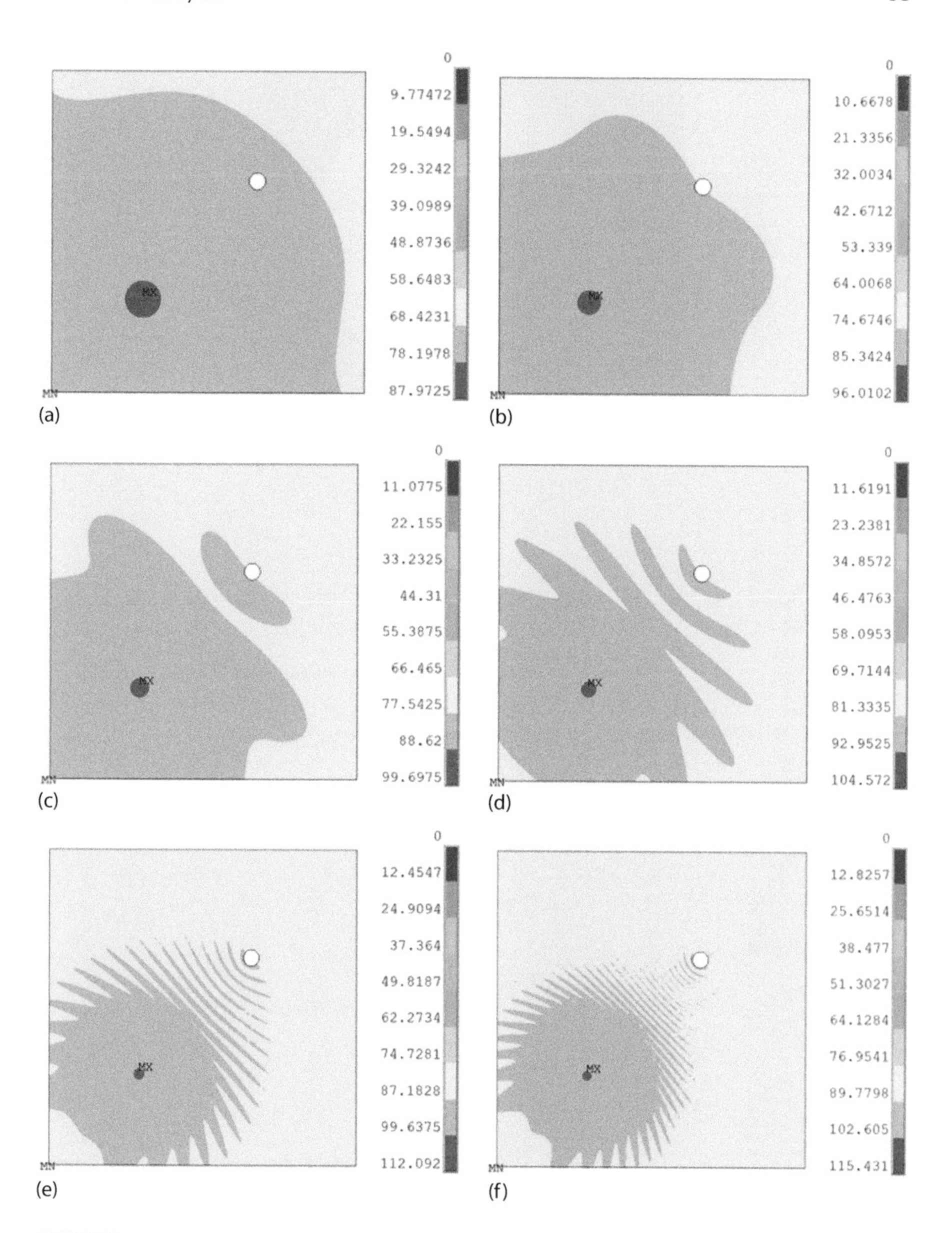

FIGURE 4.4 Acoustic pressures at different frequencies: (a) 10 Hz, (b) 30 Hz, (c) 50 Hz, (d) 100 Hz, (e) 300 Hz, and (f) 500 Hz.

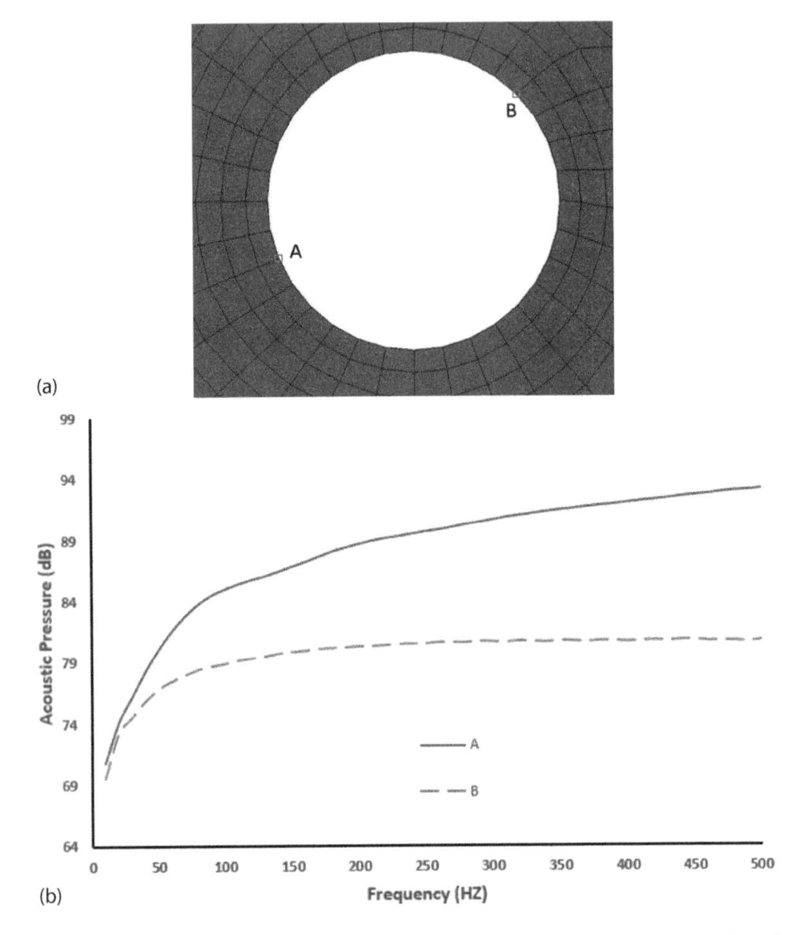

FIGURE 4.5 Variation of acoustic pressures with different frequencies: (a) locations of points A and B and (b) acoustic pressures of A and B with frequencies.

4.4.7 Summary

An acoustic finite element model was built to simulate a body in an open area under a blast. The computational results show the interaction between the incident wave and reflected wave.

REFERENCES

1. Helfer, T.M., Jordan, N.N., and Lee, R.B., "Post deployment hearing loss in U.S. Army soldiers seen at audiology clinics from April 1, 2003, through March 31, 2004," *American Journal of Audiology*, Vol. 14, 2005, pp. 161–168.
2. Cave, K.M., and Cornish, E.M., "Chandler DW: Blast injury of the ear: Clinical update from the global war on terror," *Journal of Military Medicine*, Vol. 172, 2007, pp. 726–730.

3. www.pearl-hifi.com/06_Lit_Archive/14_Books_Tech_Papers/Introduction_to_Acoustics.pdf
4. Kuttruff, H., *Acoustics an Introduction*, Taylor & Francis, New York, NY, 2007.
5. Zhang, Q., and Cen, S., *Multiphysics Modeling: Numerical Methods and Engineering Applications*, Academic Press, Cambridge, MA, 2016.
6. ANSYS help documentation in the help page of ANSYS190 Product, 2018.

5 Thermal Analysis

Heat transfer exists in the human body. Convective heat transport occurs when a significant difference exists between the temperature of the blood and the tissue through which it flows, which changes the temperatures of both the blood and the affecting tissue [1]. In addition, convection takes place when the body temperature is higher than the temperature of the environment. These phenomena are relevant to heat transfer.

Chapter 5 focuses on heat transfer—its governing equations, finite element implementation, and modeling procedure in ANSYS. The final part of Chapter 5 conducts thermal analysis of a breast tumor.

5.1 MODES OF HEAT TRANSFER

Heat flows whenever a temperature difference exists in a medium or between media. There are three heat transfer models [1] (Figure 5.1). Figure 5.1a shows that when a temperature gradient exists in a stationary medium, heat flows following the law of conduction heat transfer. As indicated in Figure 5.1b, if the temperature gradient exists between a surface and a moving fluid, convection occurs. Radiation does not need any medium to transfer heat because it is generated by electromagnetic waves, which is the third model (Figure 5.1c).

5.2 GOVERNING EQUATIONS AND FINITE ELEMENT IMPLEMENTATION

The governing equation for heat flow is given as [2]:

$$\rho c_v \frac{\partial T}{\partial t} = \nabla^{\mathrm{T}} \mathbf{k} \nabla T + \rho r \tag{5.1}$$

where:

ρ = mass density;
c_v = specific heat;
$\mathbf{k}$ = matrix of thermal conductivity;
T = temperature; and
r = energy reserve at the element per unit mass.

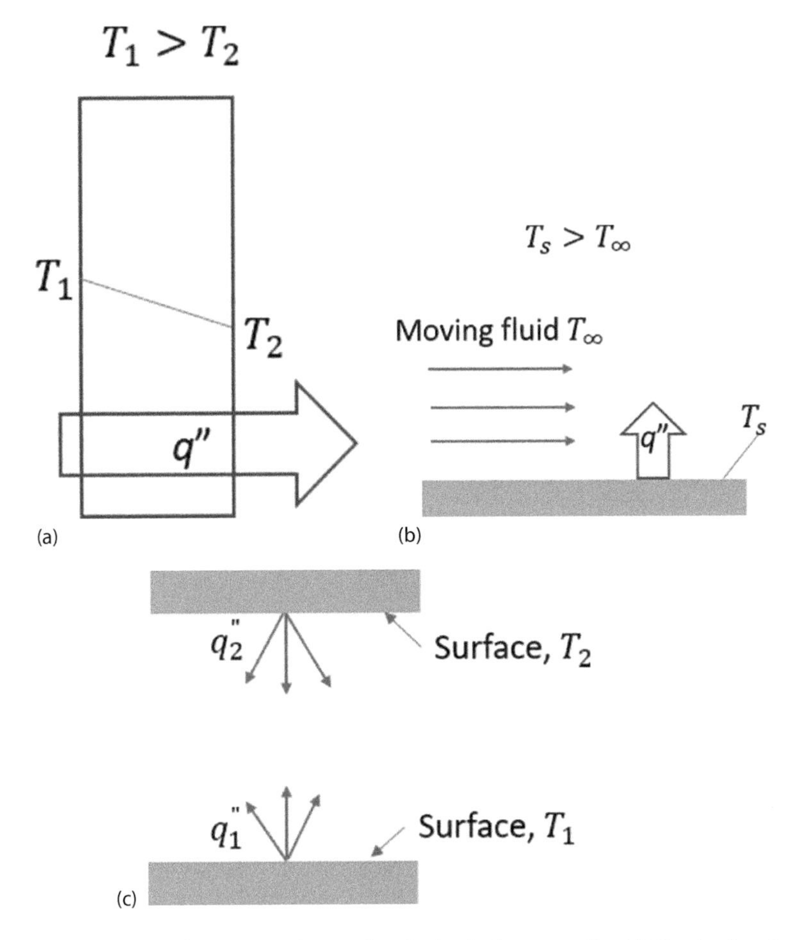

FIGURE 5.1 Conduction, convection, and radiation in heat transfer. (a) Conduction through a solid/fluid, (b) convection from a surface to a moving fluid, and (c) radiation heat exchange between surfaces. (From www.pathways.cu.edu.eg/ec/Text-PDF/Part%20A-3.pdf.)

There are three types of boundary conditions in heat flow analysis [2]:

1. Temperature on Γ_g:

$$T = T^s \text{ on } \Gamma_g \tag{5.2}$$

   where T^s is the given temperature at the boundary.

2. Heat flow on Γ_{q_1}:

$$q = -\mathbf{n}^{\mathrm{T}}\mathbf{k}\nabla T \tag{5.3}$$

   where:
   $\mathbf{n}$ = the normal direction and
   q = the heat flux at the boundary.

3. Convection surfaces over surface Γ_{q_2}:

$$q = -h_f\left(T_f - T_s\right) \tag{5.4}$$

where:

h_f = the coefficient of convective heat transfer;
T_f = the bulk temperature of the adjacent fluid; and
T_s = temperature at the surface of the model.

The finite element formula of the thermal equation is implemented by the weak form of heat flow Equation (5.1):

$$\int_V \rho c_v w_{\mathrm{T}} \frac{\partial T}{\partial t} dV + \int_V \left(\nabla w_{\mathrm{T}}\right)^{\mathrm{T}} \mathbf{k} \nabla T dV = -\int_S w_{\mathrm{T}} q dA + \int_V w_{\mathrm{T}} \rho r dV \tag{5.5}$$

where w_{T} is the test function of temperature T.

Temperature is interpolated into:

$$T = \mathbf{N}^{\mathrm{T}}\mathbf{T} \tag{5.6}$$

$$\nabla T = \mathbf{B}\mathbf{T} \tag{5.7}$$

where:

$\mathbf{N}^{\mathrm{T}}$ = shape function for temperature;
$\mathbf{B} = \partial \mathbf{N}$; and
$\mathbf{T}$ = temperature at node.

Making the testing function w_{T} as shape function and combining boundary conditions, Equations (5.2)–(5.4) with Equation (5.5) result in:

$$\mathbf{C}_e^T \dot{\mathbf{T}}^e + \left(\mathbf{K}_e^{td} + \mathbf{K}^{tc}\right)\mathbf{T}^e = \mathbf{Q}_f^{\mathrm{flux}} + \mathbf{Q}_f^{\mathrm{conv}} + \mathbf{Q}_e^g \tag{5.8}$$

where:

$$\mathbf{C}_e^T = \int_{\Omega_e} \rho c_v \mathbf{N}^{\mathrm{T}}\mathbf{N} d\Omega \tag{5.9}$$

$$\mathbf{K}_e^{td} = \int_{\Omega_e} \mathbf{B}^{\mathrm{T}}\mathbf{k}\mathbf{B} d\Omega \tag{5.10}$$

$$\mathbf{K}^{tc} = \int_{\Gamma_{q\_2}} h_f \mathbf{N}^{\mathrm{T}}\mathbf{N} d\Gamma \tag{5.11}$$

$$\mathbf{Q}_f^{\mathrm{flux}} = \int_{\Gamma_{q\_1}} \mathbf{N}^{\mathrm{T}} q d\Gamma \tag{5.12}$$

$$\mathbf{Q}_f^{\mathrm{conv}} = \int_{\Gamma_{q\_2}} h_f \mathbf{N}^{\mathrm{T}} T_f d\Gamma \tag{5.13}$$

$$\mathbf{Q}_e^g = \int_{\Omega_e} \mathbf{N}^{\mathrm{T}} \rho r d\Omega \tag{5.14}$$

Assembling Equation (5.7) into the global matrix as [2]:

$$\mathbf{C}^T\dot{\mathbf{T}} + \left(\mathbf{K}^{td} + \mathbf{K}^{tc}\right)\mathbf{T} = \mathbf{Q}^{flux} + \mathbf{Q}^{conv} + \mathbf{Q}^g \tag{5.15}$$

Specific heat matrix:

$$\mathbf{C}^T = \sum_{e=1}^{ne} \mathbf{C}_e^T \tag{5.16}$$

Diffusion conductivity matrix:

$$\mathbf{K}^{td} = \sum_{e=1}^{ne} \mathbf{K}_e^{td} \tag{5.17}$$

Convection surface conductivity matrix:

$$\mathbf{K}^{tc} = \sum_{e=1}^{ne} \mathbf{K}_e^{tc} \tag{5.18}$$

Surface heat flux vector:

$$\mathbf{Q}^{\mathrm{flux}} = \sum_f \mathbf{Q}_f^{\mathrm{flux}} \tag{5.19}$$

Convection surface heat flow vector:

$$\mathbf{Q}^{\mathrm{conv}} = \sum_f \mathbf{Q}_f^{\mathrm{conv}} \tag{5.20}$$

Heat generation vector:

$$\mathbf{Q}^g = \sum_e \mathbf{Q}_e^g \tag{5.21}$$

Here, $\sum_{e=1}^{ne}$ represents the assembly operator for an element matrix with the total *ne* elements. $\sum_f$ refers to the assembly operator for the element surface loads.

Equation (5.15) can be rewritten as:

$$\mathbf{C}^T\dot{\mathbf{T}} + \mathbf{K}^{TT}\mathbf{T} = \mathbf{Q}^T \tag{5.22}$$

where:

$$\mathbf{K}^{TT} = \mathbf{K}^{td} + \mathbf{K}^{tc} \tag{5.23}$$

and

$$\mathbf{Q}^T = \mathbf{Q}^{\text{flux}} + \mathbf{Q}^{\text{conv}} + \mathbf{Q}^g \tag{5.24}$$

Equation (5.22) was implemented in ANSYS as thermal elements like PLANE55 and SOLID70.

5.3 FINITE ELEMENT PROCEDURE OF HEAT TRANSFER IN ANSYS

The general procedure to build a thermal finite element model is listed as follows:

1. *Build the model*: The thermal model can be built in the MAPDL, ANSYS Workbench, or other CAD software.
2. *Set up the model environment*: Two-dimensional thermal elements such as PLANE55 and three-dimensional elements SOLID70 are available in ANSYS to build the thermal model.
3. *Define the material properties*: The thermal material properties, such as heat conductivity, specific heat, and density, can be defined by MP or TB commands in ANSYS.
4. *Mesh the model*: The meshing of a thermal model can be performed in ANSYS MAPDL and ANSYS workbench.
5. *Define the loadings and boundary conditions*: There are five types of thermal loadings and boundary conditions in the thermal analysis: temperature, heat flow rate, convection, heat flux, and heat generation rate. These loadings and boundary conditions are defined by the corresponding ANSYS commands.
6. *Solve the equation*: Sparse solver is one common solver for the thermal problem.
7. *Post-process the analysis*: After solution, the thermal results like temperatures, thermal fluxes, and thermal gradients can be reviewed in both POST1 and POST26 of ANSYS.

5.4 THERMAL ANALYSIS OF BREAST TUMORS

Breast cancer, which represents about 26% of all new cancer cases among women, is the most commonly diagnosed type of cancer in women [3]. If it is treated in the earliest stage, a cure rate can reach as high as 95% [4]. Because the metabolic heat production of cancerous tissue is much different from that of normal tissue [5], the development of infrared instruments has made it feasible to identify the location of the breast tumor from temperature distributions and thermal conductivities. This study conducted a thermal analysis of a breast tumor using the finite element method and addressed the relation between the temperature distribution and the location of the tumor.

5.4.1 Bio-Heat Equation

The Pennes bio-heat Equation [6]:

$$\rho_t c_p \frac{\partial T}{\partial t} = k_t \nabla^2 T + \eta_b \rho_b c_{pb} \left(T_a - T\right) + \dot{Q}_m \tag{5.25}$$

where:

k_t = thermal conductivity of the tissue;
ρ_t = density of the tissue;
c_p = specific heat of the tissue;
ρ_b = density of the blood;
c_{pb} = specific heat of the blood;
η_b = blood perfusion of the tissue;
$\dot{Q}_m$ = metabolic heat generation rate of the tissue; and
T_a = temperature of the artery.

The two terms on the right side of the above equation can be regarded as generalized source terms and it is rewritten as:

$$\dot{Q}_g = \eta_b \rho_b c_{pb} \left(T_a - T\right) + \dot{Q}_m = \eta_b \rho_b c_{pb} \left(T_e - T\right) \tag{5.26}$$

$$T_e = T_a + \frac{\dot{Q}_m}{\eta_b \rho_b c_{pb}} \tag{5.27}$$

Thus, the Pennes bio-heat equation can be expressed as:

$$\rho_t c_p \frac{\partial T}{\partial t} = k_t \nabla^2 T + \dot{Q}_g \tag{5.28}$$

Equation (5.26) states that the bio-heat source is a function of body temperature.

5.4.2 Finite Element Model

A human breast was approximated by a two-dimensional semicircle with a radius of 9 cm (Figure 5.2). A tumor was modeled as a circle with a radius of 11.5 mm and 2 cm underneath the surface (skin). The whole model was meshed by thermal element PLANE55.

5.4.3 Material Properties

The thermophysical properties of breast tissue and a tumor are listed in Table 5.1 [7].

To describe the heat generation of the normal tissue and tumor, nodes in the normal tissue and tumor were assigned with lumped thermal mass elements MASS71 with different real constants, respectively.

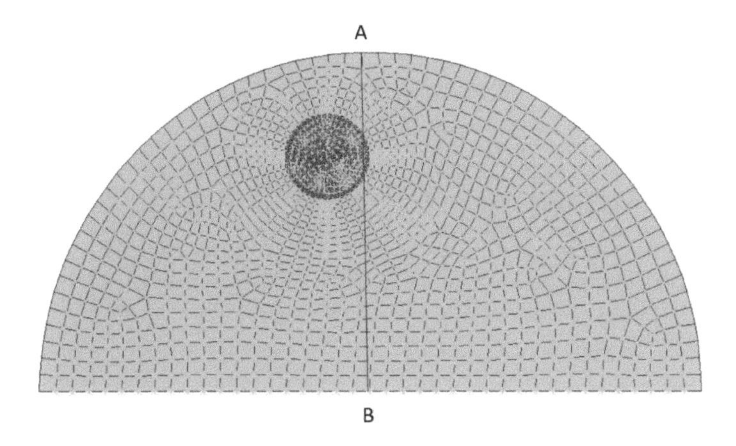

FIGURE 5.2 Finite element model of a breast tumor.

TABLE 5.1
Thermophysical Properties of Breast Tissue and Tumor

	$\rho\left(\text{kg/m}^3\right)$	$c_p\left(\text{J/kg}\cdot\text{K}\right)$	$k(\text{W/m}\cdot\text{K})$	Metabolic Heat Generation Rate $\dot{Q}_m\left(\text{W/m}^3\right)$	Blood Perfusion Rate $\eta_b\left(\text{s}^{-1}\right)$	$\frac{\dot{Q}_m}{\eta_b\rho_b c_{pb}}(°C)$
Normal tissue	920	3,000	0.42	450	0.92e–3	0.18
Tumor	1,052	3,800	0.42	29,000	0.006	1.21

The heat generation rate equation of MASS71 is expressed as [8]:

$$q(T) = A_1 + A_2T + A_3T^{A_4} + A_5T^{A_6} \tag{5.29}$$

By comparing Equation (5.26) with the heat generation rate of Equation (5.29) of MASS71, the real constants of MASS71 for the normal tissue and tumor are specified as:

```
ET,2,71,,,1,1            ! keyopt(3)=1, keyopt(4)=1
R,2,Vol_1*496.8,(35.8+273),-1
  ! vol_1 = area of normal tissue/number of nodes in normal tissue
  ! ηbρbCpb =496.8 for normal tissue
  ! Te = Ta + Qm/(ηbρbCpb) =35.6+0.18=35.78
ET,3,71,,,1,1            ! keyopt(3)=1, keyopt(4)=1
R,3,VOL_2*35978,(36.8+273),-1
! vol_2 = area of tumor/number of nodes in tumor
```

```
! ηbρbCpb = 35978 for tumor
! Te = Ta + Q̇m/(ηbρbCpb) = 35.6+1.21=36.81
```

5.4.4 Boundary Conditions

The base of the semicircle is assumed to be at adiabatic. The skin surface was exposed to a convective condition ($T_f = 20°\text{C}, h = 10\text{W/m}^2\text{K}$) (Figure 5.3). The core temperature of the body (point O) and the temperature of the arterial blood T_a were assigned as 35.78°C and 35.6°C, respectively. The initial temperature was selected as 35.78°C and 36.81°C for the normal tissues and the tumor, respectively.

5.4.5 Solution Setting

A long time (1,000 seconds) transient analysis was conducted to simulate the steady thermal state of the breast.

5.4.6 Results

Figure 5.4 plots the temperature distribution of the breast. The temperature around the tumor is the highest—about 309.8 K. The temperature away from the tumor decreases gradually and reaches 306.6 K at the skin.

The temperature along line AB is presented in Figure 5.5. It increases gradually from the skin (point A) and reaches the peak around the tumor; it then decreases away from the tumor and approaches a constant. Overall, ANSYS results match the reference [7]. In this study, the breast was simplified as a two-dimensional model. If it is modeled as three-dimensional, it should match the reference better.

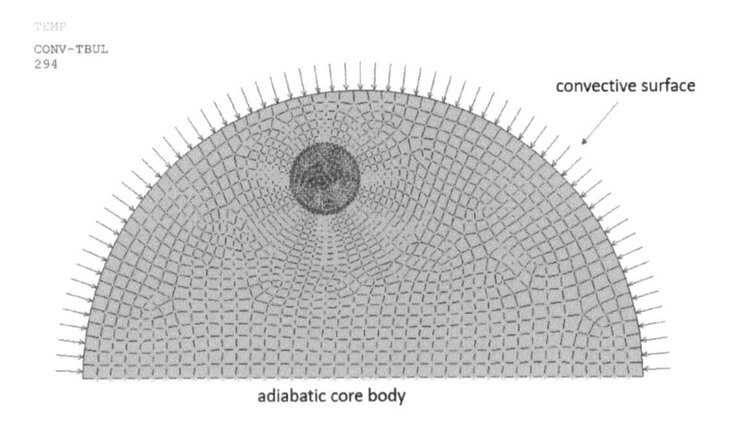

FIGURE 5.3 Boundary conditions.

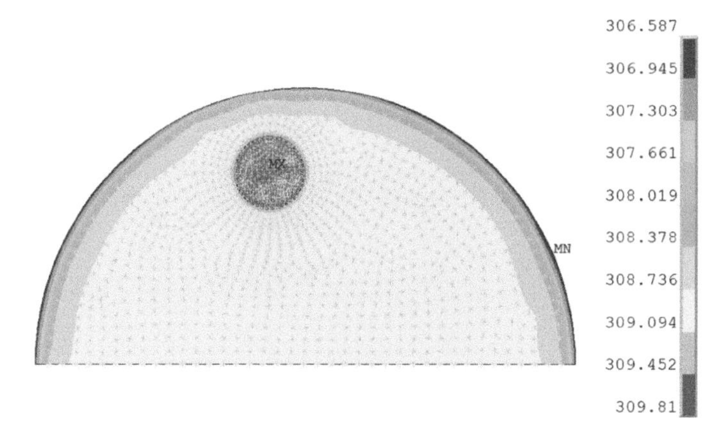

FIGURE 5.4 Temperature contour (K).

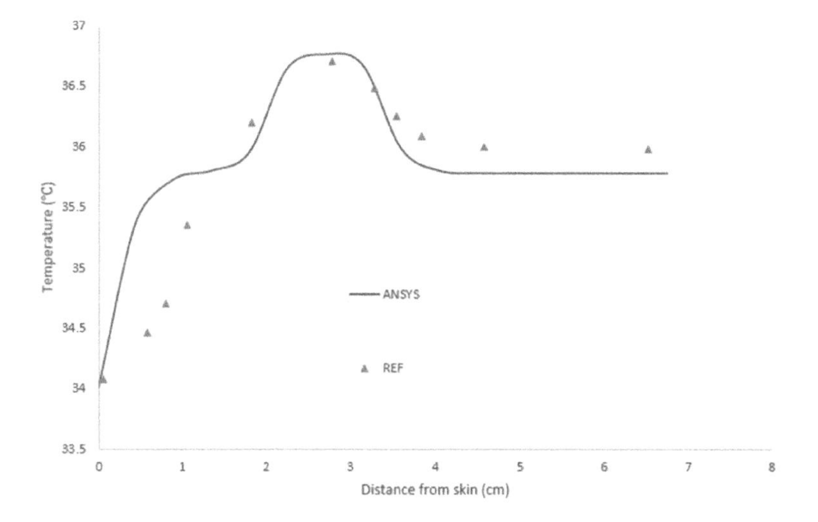

FIGURE 5.5 Temperatures along path AB.

5.4.7 Summary

A two-dimensional finite element model of the breast was created in ANSYS, and a thermal analysis of the breast tumor was performed. The results match the reference.

REFERENCES

1. www.pathways.cu.edu.eg/ec/Text-PDF/Part%20A-3.pdf.
2. Dill, E.H., *The Finite Element Method for Mechanics of Solids with ANSYS Applications*, CRC Press, Boca Raton, FL, 2011.
3. Jemal, A., Siegel, R., Ward, E., Murray, T., Xu, J., and Thun, M.J., "Cancer statistics, 2007," *A Cancer Journal for Clinicians*, Vol. 57, 2007, pp. 43–66.

4. Gamigami, P., *Atlas of Mammography: New Early Signs in Breast Cancer*, Blackwell Science, Oxford, UK, 1996.
5. Gautherie, M., "Thermopathology of breast cancer: Measurement and analysis of in vivo temperature and blood flow," *Annals of the New York Academy of Sciences*, Vol. 335, 1980, pp. 383–415.
6. Pennes, H.H., "Analysis of tissue and arterial blood temperatures in the resting human forearm," *Journal of Applied Physiology*, Vol. 1, 1948, pp. 93–122.
7. Gonzalez, F.J., "Thermal simulation of breast tumors," *Revista Mexicana De F´Isica*, Vol. 53, 2007, pp. 323–326.
8. ANSYS help documentation in the help page of product ANSYS190, 2018.

Section II

Coupling Between Two Physics Phases

In the first section, four single physics phases, including structural analysis, fluid analysis, acoustic analysis, and thermal analysis are discussed. These phases have their unique features. The second section focuses on the coupling of these phases, especially fluid structure interaction (FSI), porous media, thermal-structure coupling, and acoustic FSI. In these coupling problems, different physics phases share a common volume or interface, where all the governing equations and boundary conditions from different physical domains should be satisfied at the same time. Therefore, these couplings have their individual features and are introduced separately in Section II.

Chapter 6 discusses the general features and methods of coupling problems. Then, Chapter 7 presents FSI and its modeling procedure with an application for the study of abdominal aortic aneurysm (AAA) with two-way coupling and one-way coupling methods, respectively.

Soft tissues are biphasic with both solid and fluid phases. The governing equations of the porous media and their finite element modeling procedure are introduced in the first section of Chapter 8; the simulation of biological tissues in the confined compression test then follows.

Chapter 9 reviews acoustic FSI, including its governing equation and finite element modeling procedure in ANSYS, and presents an application for the study of the acoustic wave transmission in the ear.

Thermal-structural analysis covering the governing equation and finite element procedure, as well as the modeling of the temperature change of biological tissues under cycle loadings, are the topics for Chapter 10.

6 Introduction of Coupling Problems

Multiphysics problems cover—but are not limited to—coupling among thermal, structural, fluidic, and acoustic problems. The couplings may happen between two physics models, such as fluid-structure interaction (FSI), porous media (coupling of solid and fluid), acoustic-structural interaction (acoustic FSI), and thermal-structural analysis. Sometimes, the couplings become more complicated with more than two physics domains like the porous media thermal problem (solid + fluid + thermal).

The coupling between two physical domains may share coupling volume (Figure 6.1a) or coupling interface (Figure 6.2a). For instance, soft tissues are biphasic, in which the solid phase shares the volume with the fluid phase (Figure 6.1b). When the blood flows in the vessel, the blood shares the vessel wall with the vessel (Figure 6.2b). At the common volume or interface, all the governing equations and boundary condition from different physical domains should be satisfied simultaneously. For example, in FSI, the boundary conditions at the interface surface are controlled by the kinematic and traction coupling conditions [1]. The kinematic coupling condition requires that the fluid velocity equals the time derivative of the solid displacement at the FSI wall:

$$v_i = \frac{du_i}{dt} \tag{6.1}$$

where:
v_i = the fluid velocity and
u_i = the solid displacement at the solid boundary.

The traction coupling condition can be regarded as the stress balance between the fluid and the structure.

$$t_i^s + t_i^f = 0 \tag{6.2}$$

The numerical discretization, especially at the interface surface, significantly influences the coupling problems. When two different physical domains are meshed together, the nodal positions between the two physical meshes are coincident. Thus, the governing equations of two physical domains are solved jointly. This approach is called the monolithic approach [2] (Figure 6.3).

Unlike the monolithic approach, the partitioned approach solves two physics phases separately in sequential order using different meshing. Therefore, the nodal positions in the two physics phases do not match. Compared with the monolithic approach, the partitioned approach is very fast and efficient, although it requires much more convergences.

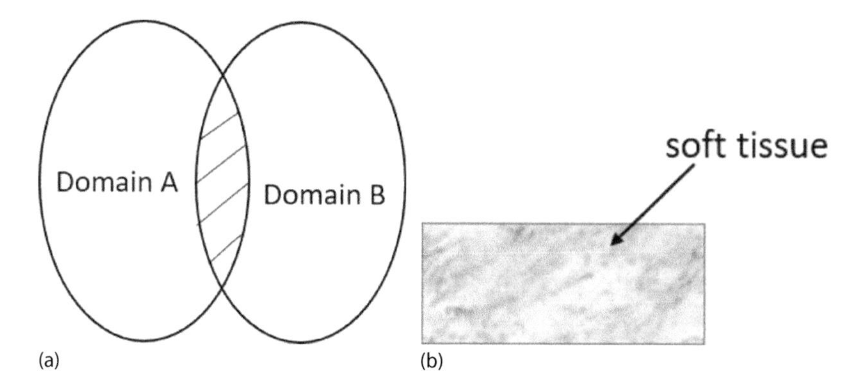

FIGURE 6.1 Coupling shares the coupling volume (a) coupling with common volume and (b) soft tissue.

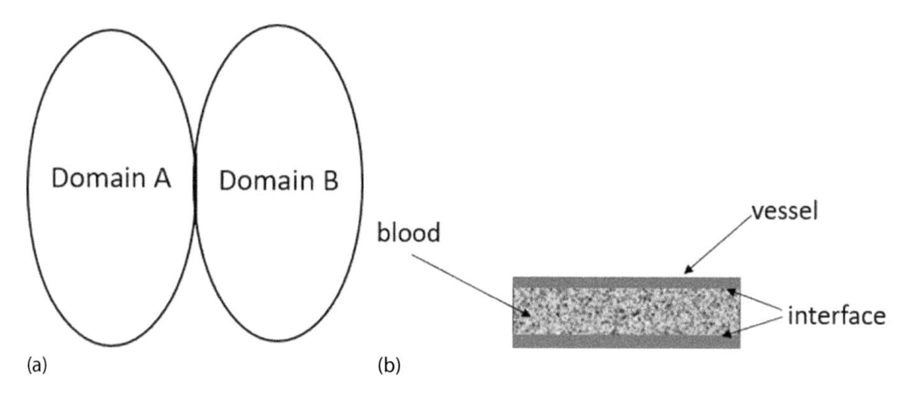

FIGURE 6.2 Coupling shares the coupling interface (a) coupling with common interface and (b) blood in vessel.

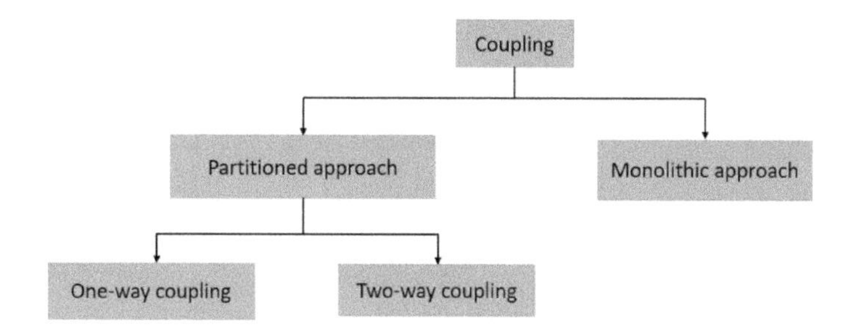

FIGURE 6.3 Coupling approaches. (From Kesti, J. and Olsson, S., *Fluid Structure Interaction Analysis on the Aerodynamic Performance of Underbody Panels*, Master's Thesis, Chalmers University of Technology, 2014.)

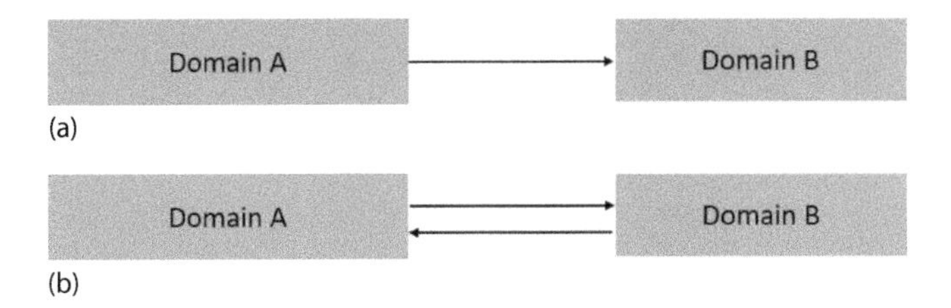

FIGURE 6.4 Data transfer between domains (a) one-way coupling and (b) two-way coupling.

Figure 6.3 illustrates that the partitioned approach is classified into two groups: one-way coupling and two-way coupling [3]. One-way coupling requires that transfer quantities are sent from one domain to another, but not in the opposite direction (Figure 6.4a). In two-way coupling, data transfer frequently between the two domains in both directions. This procedure continues in an iterative process until the convergence is reached (Figure 6.4b).

Normally, the monolithic approach and two-way coupling are used for a coupling system with a high correlation between physics models. Therefore, they are always called strong coupling. On the other hand, one-way coupling is applied for the coupling with low dependency between physical models, which is called weak coupling.

REFERENCES

1. Zienkiewicz, O.C., Taylor, R.L., and Nithiarasu, P., *The Finite Element Method for Fluid Dynamics*, Butterworth-Heinemann, Oxford, UK, 2014.
2. Kesti, J., and Olsson, S., *Fluid Structure Interaction Analysis on the Aerodynamic Performance of Underbody Panels*, Master's Thesis, Chalmers University of Technology, 2014.
3. Benra, F.K., Dohmen, H.J., Pei, J., Schuster, S., and Wan, B., "A comparison of one-way and two-way coupling methods for numerical analysis of fluid-structure interactions," *Journal of Applied Mathematics*, 2011, 16 p.

7 Fluid-Structure Interaction

In the human body, blood flows in the vessel, air comes in and out of the lung, and urine flows through the ureter. Because the soft tissues around the blood, air, and urine are deformable, an interaction between fluid and soft tissues exists. Therefore, fluid-structure interaction (FSI) as one feature of system coupling in ANSYS can be applied to study the fluid flow in the human body.

After a short introduction of two-way and one-way FSI couplings in ANSYS, Chapter 7 analyzes abdominal aortic aneurysm (AAA) with two-way and one-way coupling approaches in ANSYS Workbench, respectively.

7.1 FSI IN ANSYS

The partitioned approach is widely used for FSI simulation in ANSYS. Therefore, the two-way and one-way FSI couplings are briefly described.

7.1.1 Two-Way FSI Coupling in ANSYS

Two-way FSI coupling in ANSYS is implemented in ANSYS Workbench, in which the structural analysis and ANSYS Fluent are connected by system coupling. The overview of the coupling procedure is listed in Figure 7.1 [1]. The coupling procedure first starts in ANSYS Fluent, and the results (forces) transfer to the structural model. Then, the computation switches to the structural analysis. After computing the deformation and stresses in the structural analysis, a deformed surface is obtained. With the updated geometry, the CFD meshing is morphed to adjust for the deformation (Figure 7.2). At the end of the sequence, convergence criteria are checked to see if the pressure field and the deformation become stable between each iteration. This procedure repeats until convergence or maximum iterations are reached.

A finite element model for the two-way FSI coupling in ANSYS is composed of three parts (Figure 7.3): structural analysis, ANSYS Fluent, and system coupling. The structural model and fluent model are built following the procedure listed in Chapters 2 and 3, respectively. Both the structural model and fluent model should specify individual FSI components in each model, and the data transfer between the FSI components is defined in the system coupling.

7.1.2 One-Way FSI Coupling in ANSYS

One-way FSI coupling in ANSYS is relatively simple (Figure 7.4). After the fluid solution, the pressures transfer to the solid through the FSI wall. Then, the structural analysis is performed (Figure 7.5). After the structural solution, the stresses and

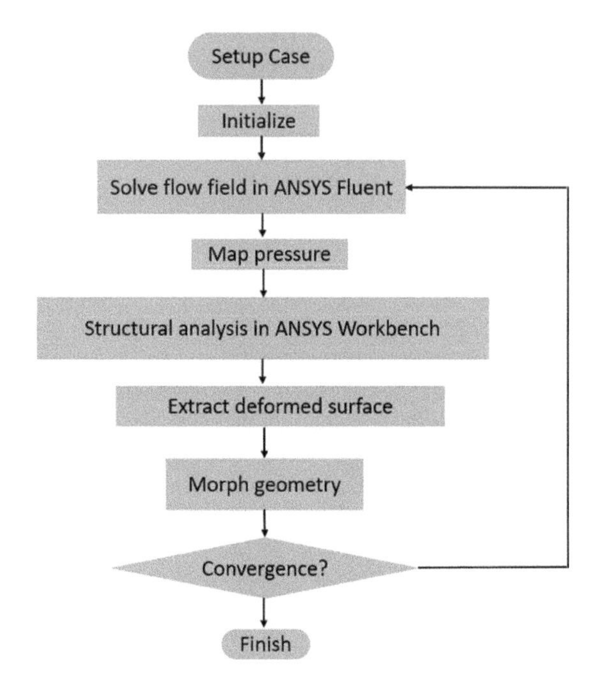

FIGURE 7.1 Flow chart of two-way FSI in ANSYS. (From Kesti, J. and Olsson, S., *Fluid Structure Interaction Analysis on the Aerodynamic Performance of Underbody Panels*, Master's Thesis, Chalmers University of Technology, 2014.)

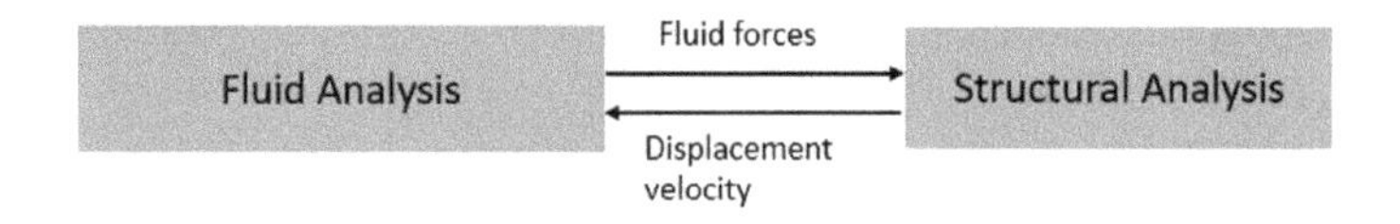

FIGURE 7.2 Data transfer in two-way FSI.

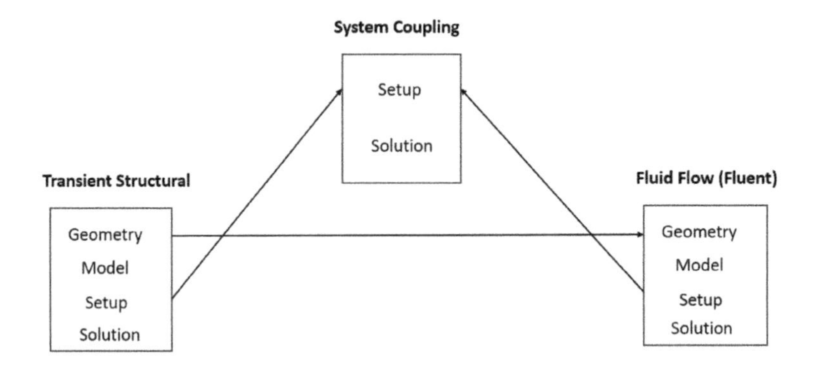

FIGURE 7.3 Schematic of two-way FSI in ANSYS Workbench.

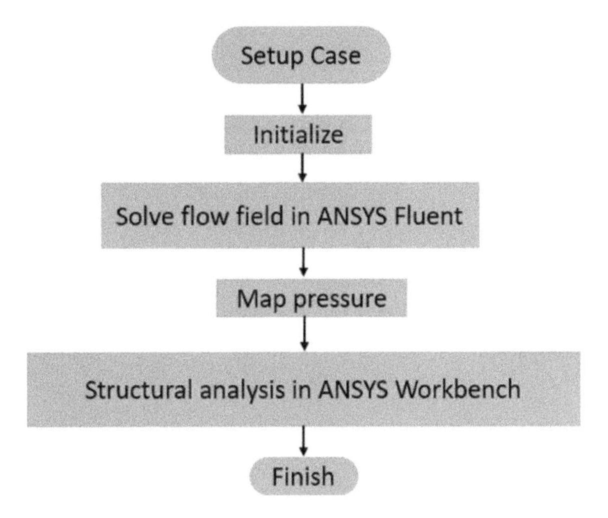

FIGURE 7.4 Flow chart of one-way FSI in ANSYS.

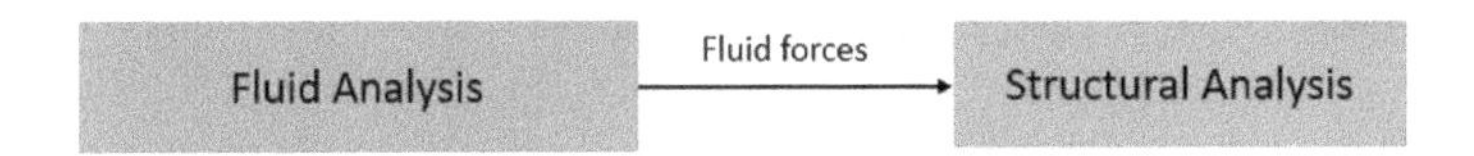

FIGURE 7.5 Data transfer in one-way FSI.

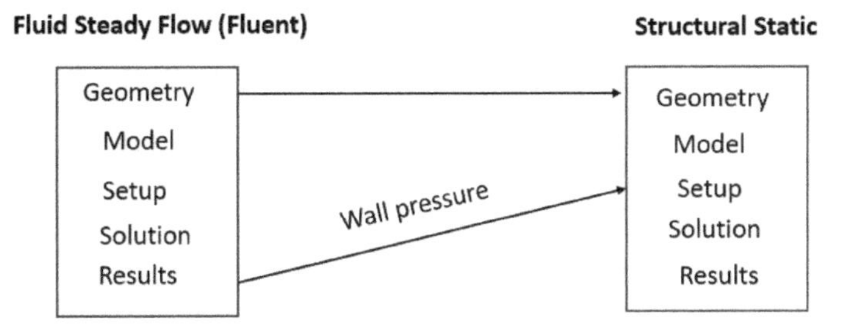

FIGURE 7.6 Schematic of one-way FSI in ANSYS Workbench.

the deformation are obtained. Unlike two-way FSI coupling, one-way FSI coupling completes in one iteration.

A finite element model for the one-way FSI coupling in ANSYS comprises structural analysis and ANSYS Fluent (Figure 7.6). In the model, pressures obtained in ANSYS Fluent should be defined as the loading of the structural analysis.

7.2 STUDY OF ABDOMINAL AORTIC ANEURYSM BY TWO-WAY FSI

Nearly two million Americans suffer from AAA disease, and the rate of occurrence keeps growing. The aneurysm diameter increases at the rate of around 0.4 cm/year until rupture (Figure 7.7), and the AAA rupture is the thirteenth most common

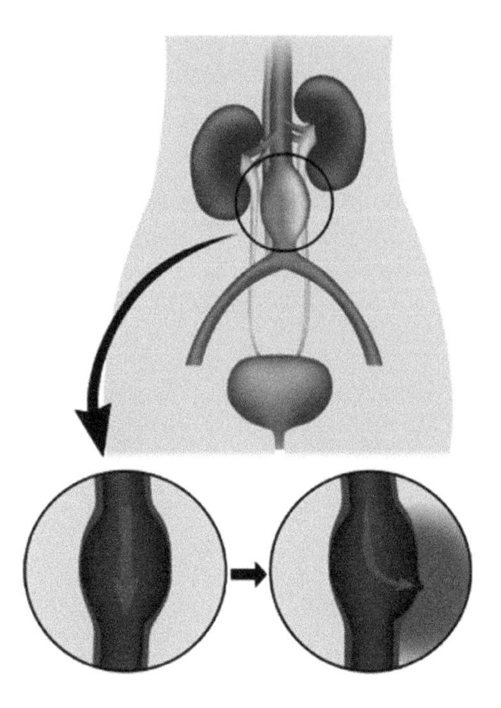

FIGURE 7.7 Abdominal aortic aneurysm (Alila© 123RF.com).

cause of death in the United States [2]. Currently, the transverse dimension of the aneurysm—5 cm—is regarded as the primary indicator for a potential rupture in the clinical management of AAA patients. However, some clinical cases show that some AAAs ruptured at a size less than 5 cm, and other AAAs grew to 8 cm without rupture. Thus, some studies suggest that the strength of the wall tissue of AAAs can be the indictor of an AAA rupture. Therefore, an intensive study of the wall stress of AAA has been conducted [3–13], which can be classified into two categories: (1) study the wall stress of AAAs using static pressures on the wall and (2) study AAAs by fully coupled FSI that simultaneously computes the flow and pressure fields in the aneurysm with the wall stresses. Obviously, including both the dynamics of blood flow and the wall motion response is a more accurate way to model the aneurysm. As a result, a fully coupling study of AAAs was conducted in ANSYS Workbench.

7.2.1 System Coupling Implementation

The fully coupling study implemented in ANSYS Workbench consists of three parts: (1) structural transient analysis, (2) transient fluent analysis, and (3) system coupling (Figure 7.3). The structural analysis shares the geometry with the fluent analysis, and the solution setting of the structural analysis and the fluid analysis is associated with the system coupling. The details of the three parts are given in the following.

7.2.1.1 Structural Analysis

7.2.1.1.1 Geometry and Meshing

A half-aneurysm model was generated with the CAD software SpaceClaim, with a diameter of 2 cm at the inlet and outlet sections and a maximum diameter of 6 cm at the midsection of the AAA sac (Figure 7.8). The asymmetry of the model is governed by the β parameter defined by [9]:

$$\beta = r / R \tag{7.1}$$

where r and R are the radii measured at the midsection of the AAA sac as shown in Figure 7.8b.

In this model, β was selected as 0.6.

The AAA wall was assumed with uniform thickness 1.5 mm. The whole model was meshed with SHELL181.

7.2.1.1.2 Material Properties

The blood vessel was assumed as linear elastic with Young's modulus 2.7 MPa and Poisson's ratio 0.45.

7.2.1.1.3 Loading and Boundary Conditions

Two ends of the blood vessel were constrained, and the surface of the AAA wall was specified as the system coupling (Figure 7.9).

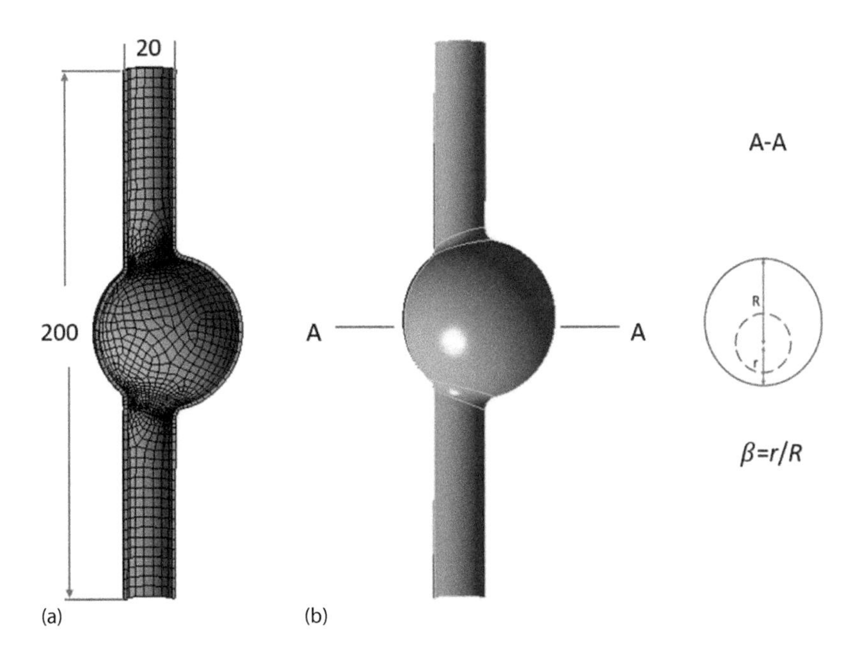

FIGURE 7.8 Finite element model of abdominal aortic aneurysm: (a) finite element model (all dimensions in mm) and (b) cross section of the model.

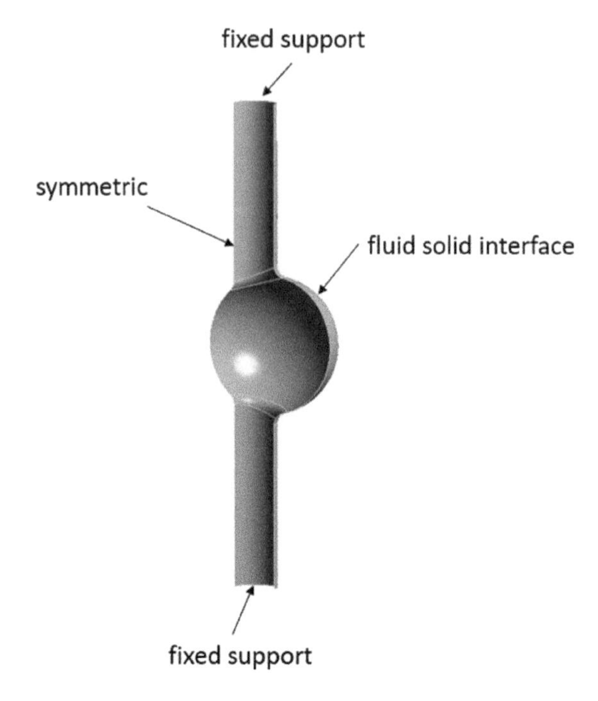

FIGURE 7.9 Loadings and boundary conditions of AAA.

7.2.1.1.4 Solution Setting

Transient analysis was performed in 3 seconds, around three cycles of the pulsatile pressure. Each time step was fixed to be 0.05 seconds.

The above modeling procedure in ANSYS Workbench can be found in the online video:

www.feabea.net/models/mech.mp4

7.2.1.2 CFD Fluent Analysis

7.2.1.2.1 Geometry and Meshing

The fluid domain was meshed in ANSYS Workbench, in which the part close to the boundary was meshed finer due to the boundary layer of fluid (Figure 7.10).

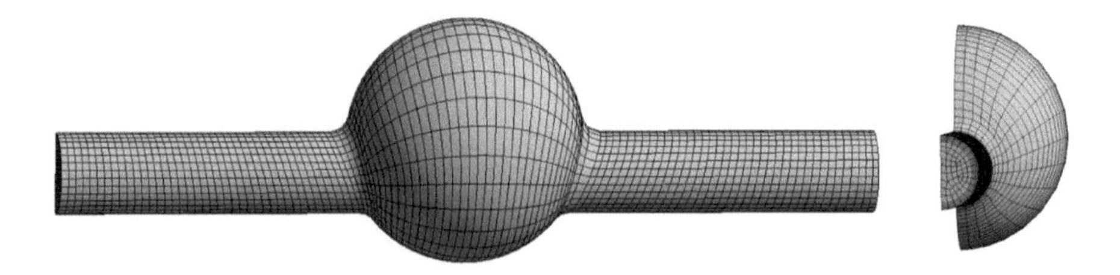

FIGURE 7.10 Mesh of AAA in ANSYS fluent.

7.2.1.2.2 Material Properties

The density and dynamic viscosity of the blood were defined as 1050 kg/m^3 and 0.00385 Pa.s, respectively.

7.2.1.2.3 Boundary Conditions

The time-dependent fully developed velocity profile on the inlet is represented by:

$$v(t,x,y) = u(t)\left(\frac{r^2 - x^2 - y^2}{r^2}\right) \quad (7.2)$$

where:

$u(t)$ = time-dependent velocity from the experiment data (Figure 7.11) [10],
r = the radius of the inlet, and
x and y = the coordinates in x and y directions.

Equation (7.2) was implemented in the udf (Appendix A).

The pressure at the outlet was given as 10,000 Pa.

The wall was defined as system coupling (Figure 7.12), and the blood as deformable.

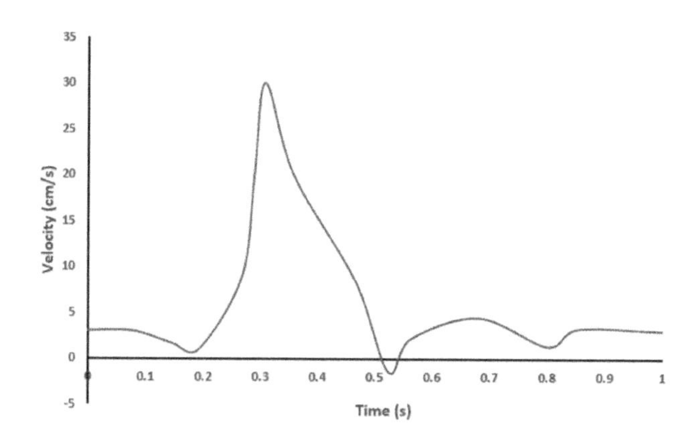

FIGURE 7.11 In vivo luminal pulsatile velocity.

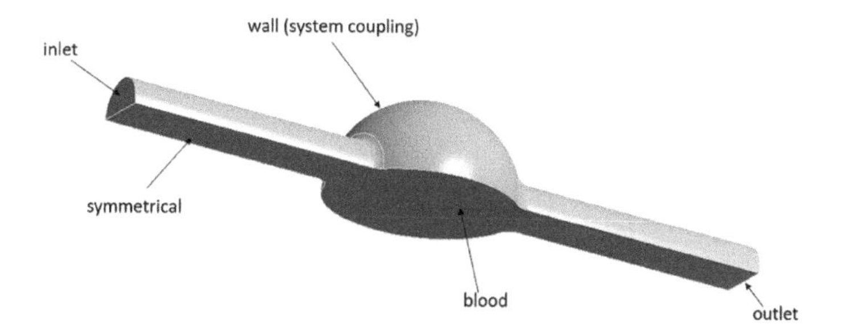

FIGURE 7.12 Boundary conditions of AAA in two-way FSI.

7.2.1.2.4 Solution Setting

The flow was defined as laminar [10]. The whole time was set to be 3 seconds with time step 0.05 seconds, which is the same as that of structural analysis.

The above modeling procedure in ANSYS Fluent can be found in the online videos:

www.feabea.net/models/cfd_meshing.mp4
www.feabea.net/models/cfd.mp4

7.2.1.3 System Coupling

The wall of the blood vessel in the structural analysis and the wall of the blood fluid in the CFD analysis built the data transfer in the system coupling. In addition, the computational time and time step were assigned as 3 and 0.05 seconds, respectively, which is the same as the structural analysis and CFD analysis. The modeling procedure of the system coupling in ANSYS Workbench can be found in the online video:

www.feabea.net/models/coupling.mp4

7.2.2 Results

The computation got the convergence, and the convergence information was given in Figure 7.13.

Figures 7.14 and 7.15 illustrate the deformation and vM stresses of the blood vessel, respectively, which indicate that the results of the first second are affected by the initial conditions, and the results of the next two seconds are nearly the same.

Convergence information

```
+=============================================================================+
| COUPLING STEP = 60                                 SIMULATION TIME = 3.0 [s] |
+-----------------------------------------------------------------------------+
|                                       |      Source           Target        |
+-----------------------------------------------------------------------------+
+-----------------------------------------------------------------------------+
|                           COUPLING ITERATION = 13                            |
+-----------------------------------------------------------------------------+
| Transient Structural                  |                                      |
|   Interface: interface-1              |                                      |
|     Force                             |            Converged                 |
|       RMS Change                      |      9.75E-08         8.35E-08       |
|       Values Sum x                    |      3.89E-05        -4.94E-04       |
|       Values Sum y                    |      1.08E-03         6.40E-04       |
|       Values Sum z                    |     -6.10E+01        -6.10E+01       |
+-----------------------------------------------------------------------------+
| Fluid Flow (Fluent)                   |                                      |
|   Interface: interface-1              |                                      |
|     Incremental Displacement          |            Converged                 |
|       RMS Change                      |      1.05E-02         8.79E-03       |
|       Values Average x                |     -2.74E-08        -2.20E-08       |
|       Values Average y                |      1.26E-08         2.34E-08       |
|       Values Average z                |      4.21E-08         2.54E-08       |
+-----------------------------------------------------------------------------+
| Participant convergence status        |                                      |
|   Transient Structural                |            Converged                 |
|   Fluid Flow (Fluent)                 |            Converged                 |
+=============================================================================+
```

FIGURE 7.13 Convergence information of AAA during two-way FSI calculation.

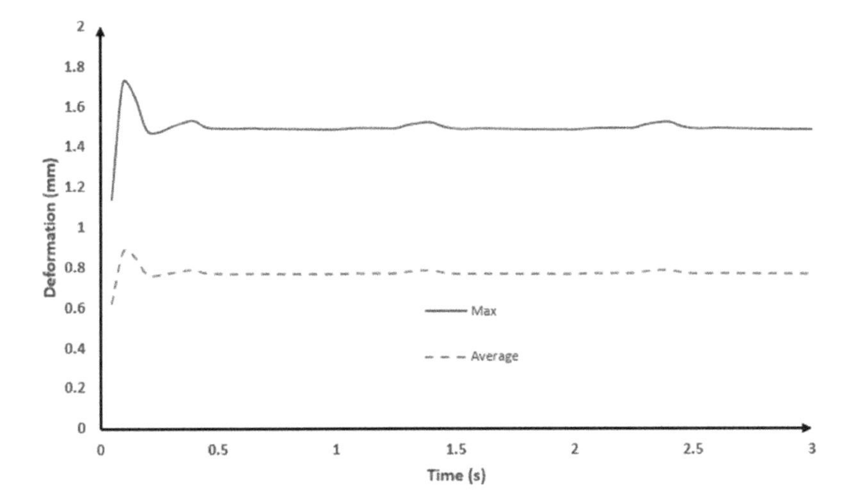

FIGURE 7.14 Deformation of AAA with time in two-way FSI.

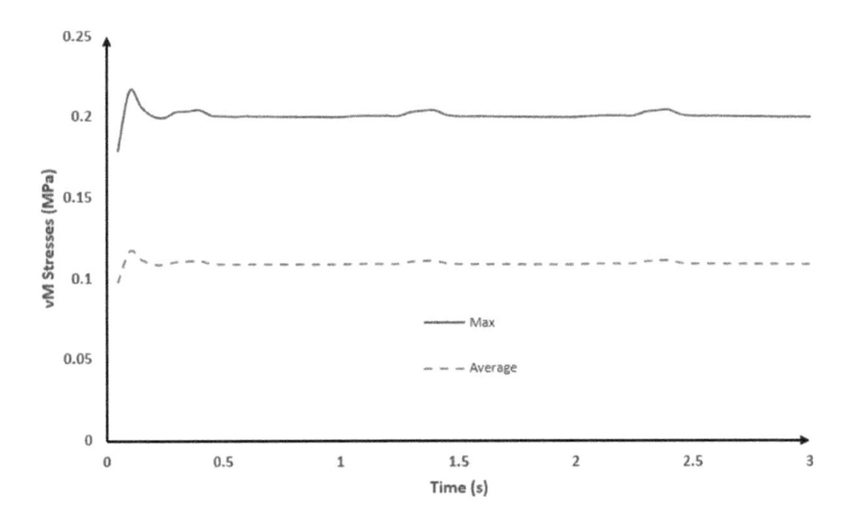

FIGURE 7.15 vM stresses of AAA with time in two-way FSI.

The results of the third second show that the maximum deformation and stress occur at time 2.4 seconds. Therefore, the deformation with maximum deformation 1.52 mm is shown in Figure 7.16, and the vM stresses with a peak value 0.204 MPa are given in Figure 7.17. At time 2.4 seconds, the pressures on the wall are plotted in Figure 7.18 and the velocity contour in Figure 7.19.

For comparison, a static analysis was performed (Figure 7.20) [14]. Figures 7.21 and 7.22 show the results of deformation (maximum value 2.39 mm) and stresses (maximum value 0.21 MPa).

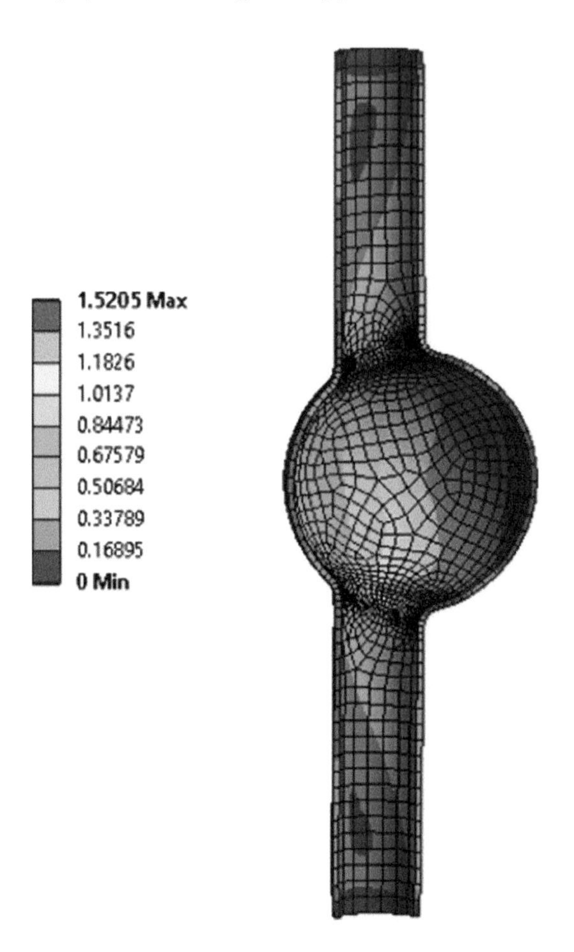

FIGURE 7.16 Deformation of AAA in two-way FSI at time $t = 2.4$ seconds (mm).

7.2.3 Discussion

A fully coupling FSI was performed to study AAAs. The computation got the convergence. The results show that the first cycle was affected by the initial conditions. The second cycle became stable.

A comparison of the FSI results with the static results shows that the peak value of the deformation changes from 1.52 mm of FSI to 2.39 mm of static analysis, more than a 50% difference, although the maximum stress is almost the same for both cases. The big difference in the deformation results confirms the necessity of a FSI analysis for modeling AAAs.

This study selected the computational time 3 seconds with time step 0.05 seconds for structural analysis, fluid analysis, and system coupling. The same time and time step make these analyses perform simultaneously, including data transfer between the FSI interface.

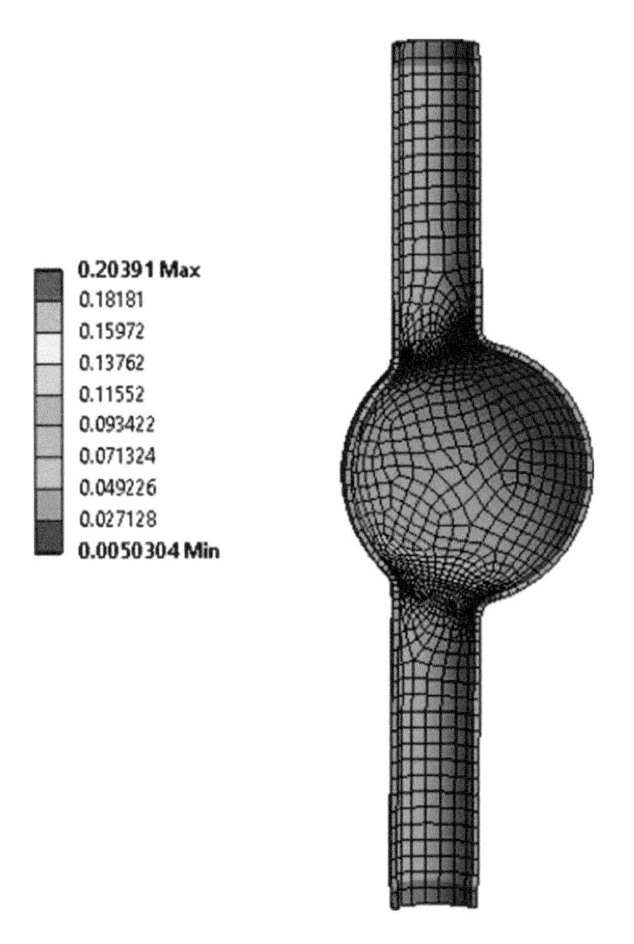

FIGURE 7.17 vM stress contour of AAA in two-way FSI at time t = 2.4 seconds (MPa).

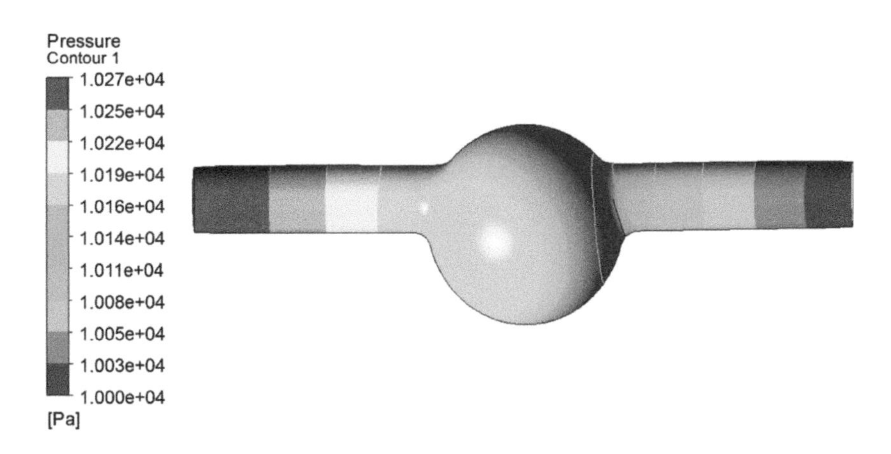

FIGURE 7.18 Wall pressure in two-way FSI at t = 2.4 seconds.

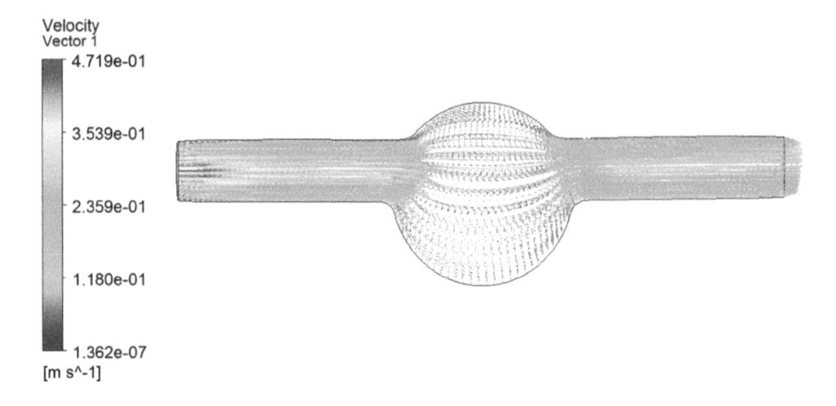

FIGURE 7.19 Blood velocity contour in two-way FSI at $t = 2.4$ seconds.

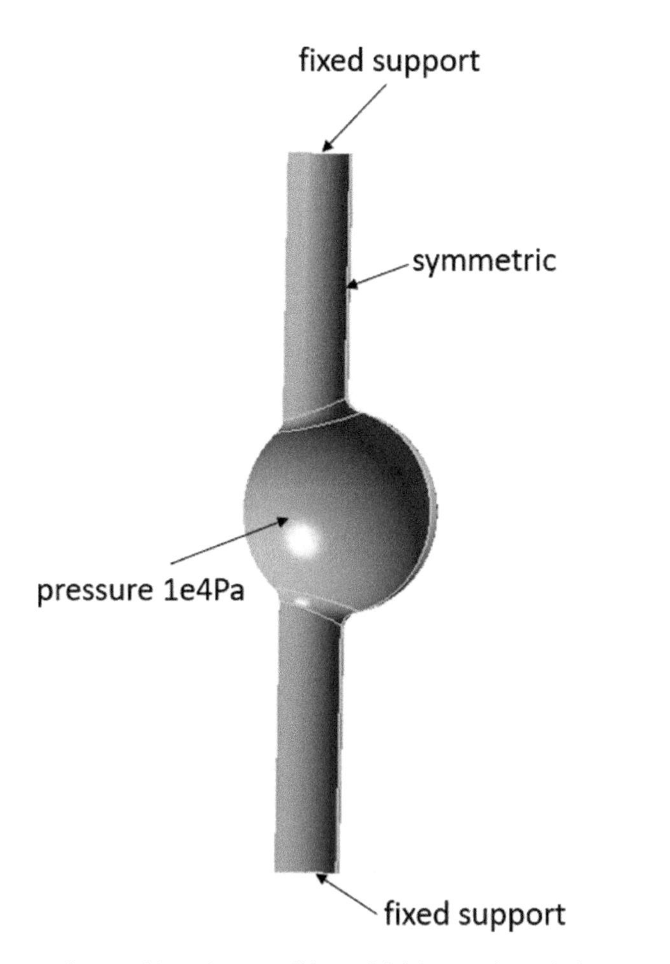

FIGURE 7.20 Loadings and boundary conditions of AAA at static analysis.

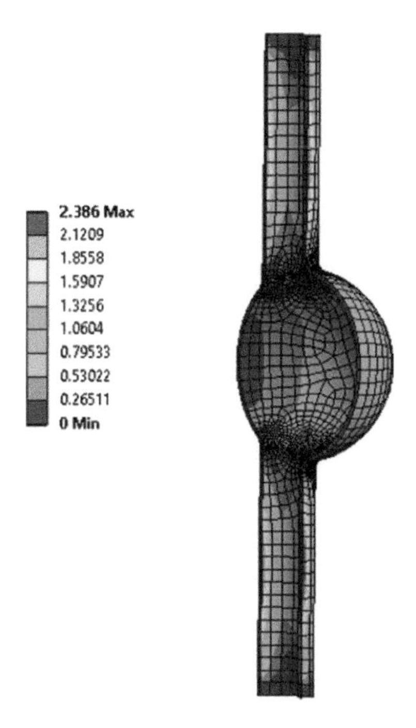

FIGURE 7.21 Deformation of AAA at static analysis (mm).

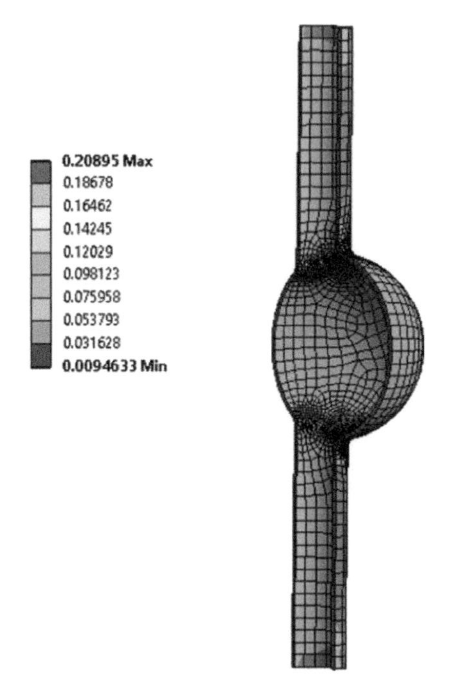

FIGURE 7.22 vM stress contour of AAA at static analysis (MPa).

7.2.4 Summary

A study of AAAs was performed in ANSYS Workbench with fully coupling FSI. The computation reached convergence, and the maximum deformation was more than 50% different from that by the static analysis.

7.3 STUDY OF AAA BY ONE-WAY COUPLING

The last section introduces the study of AAAs by fully coupling. The obtained results are much different from those in the static study, especially in the deformation of AAAs. However, fully coupling requires the data conveying between the structural analysis and the fluid analysis, and it takes many iterations to reach convergence. Therefore, fully coupling is time-consuming. To save the computational time, the one-way coupling approach was applied to study AAAs here.

7.3.1 One-Way Coupling Implementation

Unlike fully coupling, one-way coupling consists of two parts: (1) CFD fluent analysis in the steady state and (2) static structural analysis (Figure 7.6). One-way coupling is implemented as follows. First, conduct the CFD fluent analysis. Then, transfer the obtained pressures on the wall of fluid domain to the structural analysis and complete the static structural analysis. Both analyses are simply introduced in the following.

7.3.1.1 CFD Fluent Analysis

The fully developed velocity profile on the inlet is represented by:

$$v(t,x,y) = u\left(\frac{r^2 - x^2 - y^2}{r^2}\right) \tag{7.3}$$

where:

u = 0.48 m/s [10],
r = the radius of the inlet, and
x and y = the coordinates in x and y directions.

Equation (7.3) was implemented in the following udf:

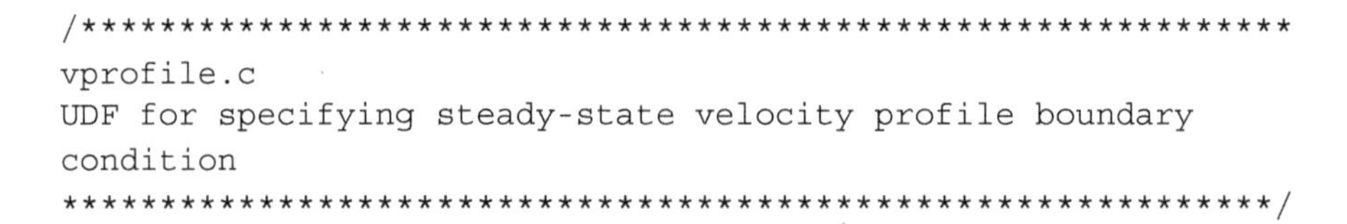

```
/*****************************************************************
vprofile.c
UDF for specifying steady-state velocity profile boundary
condition
*****************************************************************/
```

```
#include "udf.h"
DEFINE_PROFILE(inlet_x_velocity, thread, position)
{
 real x[ND_ND]; /* this will hold the position vector */
 real r, d;
 face_t f;
 r = 0.01; /* inlet height in m */
 begin_f_loop(f,thread)
 {
  F_CENTROID(x, f, thread);1
d = ((x[0]+0.0079)*(x[0]+0.0079)+x[2]*x[2])/r/r;
/* non-dimensional d coordinate */
  F_PROFILE(f, thread, position) = 0.48*(1.0-d);
 }
 end_f_loop(f, thread)
}
```

The CFD analysis was performed in ANSYS Fluent in the following steps:

1. build the geometry and meshing as done in the previous section;
2. define simulation as a steady state;
3. specify the flow as laminar;
4. define the wall in the fluid domain as system coupling [1];
5. specify density 1050 kg/m^3 and dynamic viscosity 0.00385 Pa.s in the material properties;
6. apply the velocity at the inlet by Equation (7.3) and the pressure at the outlet as 10,000 Pa; and
7. run the flow simulation.

7.3.1.2 Static Structural Analysis

The structural analysis was completed in ANSYS Workbench in the following steps:

1. build the geometry and meshing as done in the previous section;
2. define material properties of the blood vessel as done in the previous section;
3. apply constraints on both ends of the blood vessel and specify the pressure loading from the system coupling of the fluid computation [15]; and
4. run the structural simulation.

7.3.2 Results

Figure 7.23 illustrates the pressures of the whole fluid field varying from 9,998 Pa to 10,050 Pa. The velocities of the whole fluid field are plotted in Figure 7.24 with a

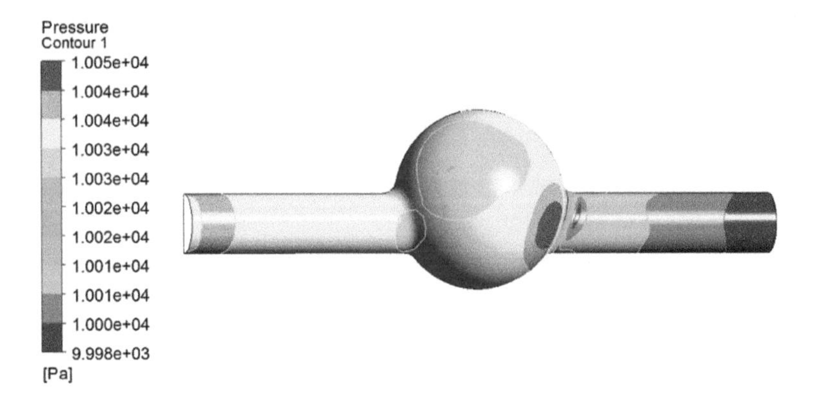

FIGURE 7.23 Pressure contour of AAA in one-way FSI.

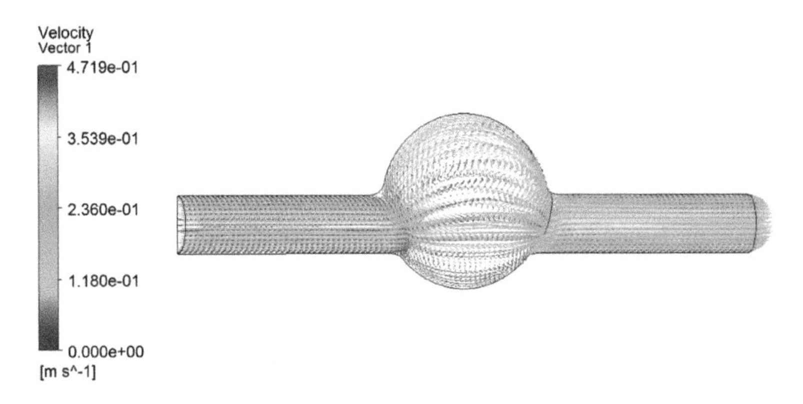

FIGURE 7.24 Velocity contour of AAA in one-way FSI.

peak value 0.47 m/s. Deformation with a maximum value 2.39 mm is presented in Figure 7.25, and vM stresses with a peak value 0.21 MPa are shown in Figure 7.26. Comparing the results with those in the previous section, the results of one-coupling are close to those of the static analysis.

7.3.3 Discussion

One-way coupling of AAAs was conducted in ANSYS Workbench. The results of the fluid analysis were considered as the loading of the static structural analysis. This one-way coupling did not consider the effect of the deformation of the blood vessel on the fluid field.

The advantage of one-way coupling over the fully coupling is saving the computational time. The computational time in this section is around a few seconds, unlike the 30 minutes of the last section. However, the results of one-way coupling are close to those by the static analysis and far from those by the fully coupling.

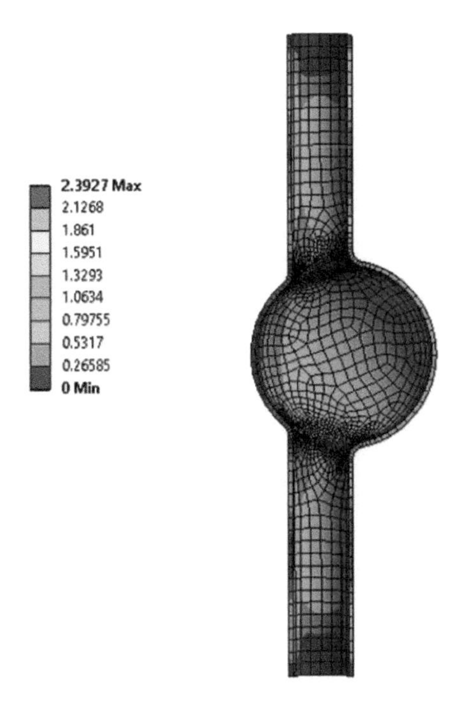

FIGURE 7.25 Deformation of AAA in one-way FSI (mm).

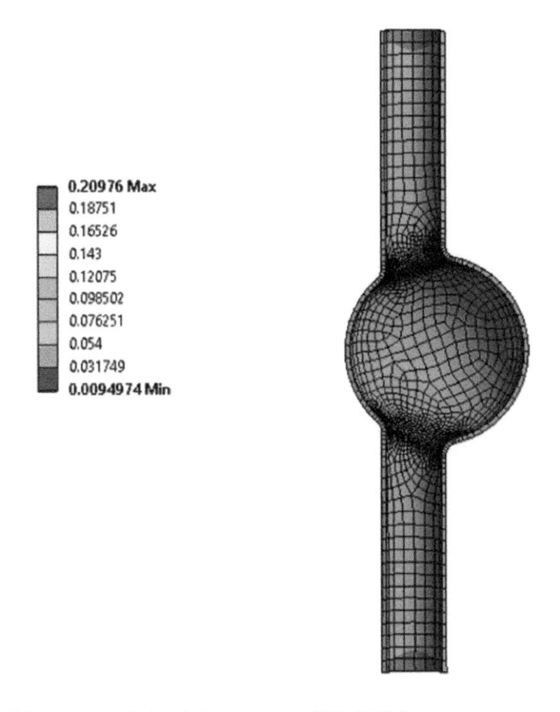

FIGURE 7.26 vM stresses of AAA in one-way FSI (MPa).

7.3.4 Summary

A study of AAAs in ANSYS Workbench was completed using one-way coupling. This approach saves much computational time, but the obtained results are close to those by the static analysis and far from those by the fully coupling.

REFERENCES

1. Kesti, J., and Olsson, S., *Fluid Structure Interaction Analysis on the Aerodynamic Performance of Underbody Panels*, Master's Thesis, Chalmers University of Technology, 2014.
2. Patel, M.I., Hardman, D.T.A., Fisher, C.M., and Appleberg, M., "Current views on the pathogenesis of abdominal aortic aneurysms," *Journal of the American College of Surgeons*, Vol. 181, 1985, pp. 371–382.
3. Di Martino, E.S., Bohra, A., Vande Geest, J.P., Gupta, N., Makaroun, M., and Vorp, D.A., "Biomechanical properties of ruptured versus electively repaired abdominal aortic aneurysm wall tissue," *Journal of Vascular Surgery*, Vol. 43, 2006, pp. 570–576.
4. Raghavan, M., Kratzberg, J., and da Silva, E.S., "Heterogeneous, variable wall-thickness modeling of a ruptured abdominal aortic aneurysm," *Proceedings of the 2004 International Mechanical Engineering Congress and R&D Expo IMECE2004*, 2004.
5. Raghavan, M.L., Vorp, D.A., Federle, M.P., Makaroun, M.S., and Webster, M.W., "Wall stress distribution on three-dimensionally reconstructed models of human abdominal aortic aneurysm," *Journal of Vascular Surgery*, Vol. 31, 2000, pp. 760–769.
6. Vorp, D.A., Raghavan, M.L., and Webster, M.W., "Mechanical wall stress in abdominal aortic aneurysm: Influence of diameter and asymmetry, "*Journal of Vascular Surgery*, Vol. 27, 1998, pp. 632–639.
7. Wilson, K.A., Lee, A.J., Hoskins, P.R., Fowkes, F.G.R., Ruckley, C.V., and Bradbury, A.W., "The relationship between aortic wall distensibility and rupture of infrarenal abdominal aortic aneurysm," *Journal of Vascular Surgery*, Vol. 37, 2003, pp. 112–117.
8. Raghavan, M.L., Kratzberg, J., Castro de Tolosa, E.M., Hanaoka, M.M., Walker, P., and da Silva, E.S., "Regional distribution of wall thickness and failure properties of human abdominal aortic aneurysm," *Journal of Biomechanics*, Vol. 39, 2006, pp. 3010–3016.
9. Scotti, C.M., Jimenez, J., Muluk, S.C., and Finol, E.A., "Wall stress and flow dynamics in abdominal aortic aneurysms: Finite element analysis vs. fluid-structure interaction," *Computer Methods in Biomechanics and Biomedical Engineering*, Vol. 11, 2008, pp. 301–322.
10. Scotti, C.M., Shkolnik, A.D., Muluk, S., and Finol, E.A., "Fluid–structure interaction in abdominal aortic aneurysms: Effects of asymmetry and wall thickness," *Biomedical Engineering Online*, Vol. 5, 2005, p. 64.
11. Raut, S., Chandra, S., Shum, J., Washington, C.B., Muluk, S.C., Finol, E.A., and Rodriguez, J.F., "Biological, geometric and biomechanical factors influencing abdominal aortic aneurysm rupture risk: A comprehensive review," *Recent Patents on Medical Imaging*, Vol. 3, 2013, pp. 44–59.
12. Ruiz de, G.S., Antón, R., Cazón, A., Larraona, G.S., and Finol, E.A., "Anisotropic abdominal aortic aneurysm replicas with biaxial material characterization," *Medical Engineering & Physics*, Vol. 38, 2016, pp. 1505–1512.

13. Ruiz de, G.S., Cazón, A., Antón, R., and Finol, E.A., "The relationship between surface curvature and abdominal aortic aneurysm wall stress," *Journal of Biomechanical Engineering*, Vol. 139, 2017, doi:10.1115/1.4036826.
14. Yang, Z., *Finite Element Analysis for Biomedical Engineering Applications*, CRC Press, Boca Raton, FL, 2019.
15. ANSYS help documentation in the help page of product ANSYS190.

8 Modeling of Porous Media

Soft tissues are regarded as porous media because they are comprised of solid and water components. For example, the nucleus pulposus, a mucoprotein gel in the center of the intervertebral disc, consists of a great amount of sulfated glycosaminoglycans in a network of type II collagen. The water in the nucleus varies from 90% at birth to 80% in a young adult, and keeps decreasing with age [1]. Therefore, it is appropriate to model the soft tissues as porous media.

After introducing the governing equations and finite element modeling procedure of porous media, Chapter 8 simulates the biological tissue in the confined compression test.

8.1 GOVERNING EQUATIONS FOR POROUS MEDIA

Porous media is biphasic with both the solid and fluid phases. Figure 8.1 shows a point of the biphasic material, including the solid phase and fluid phase. Both phases interact by pore pressure p. Therefore, the solid phase is governed by:

$$\nabla \cdot \left(\sigma'' - \alpha p \mathbf{I}\right) + \mathbf{b} = \rho \ddot{\mathbf{u}} \tag{8.1}$$

where:

σ'' = the effective stress of the solid phase
$\mathbf{b}$ = body force
α = Biot coefficient

The fluid phase follows Darcy's law. Thus,

$$\mathbf{q} = -k\nabla p \tag{8.2}$$

where $\mathbf{q}$ is the fluid flux.

Based on the mass conservation, the storage due to compressibility of the solid and of the fluid should be equal to the dilation of the solid and of the fluid [2]. Thus,

$$\nabla \cdot \mathbf{q} + \alpha \dot{\varepsilon}_V + \frac{\dot{p}}{Q^*} = 0 \tag{8.3}$$

where:

ε_V = volumetric strain of the solid skeleton
Q^* = compressibility parameter

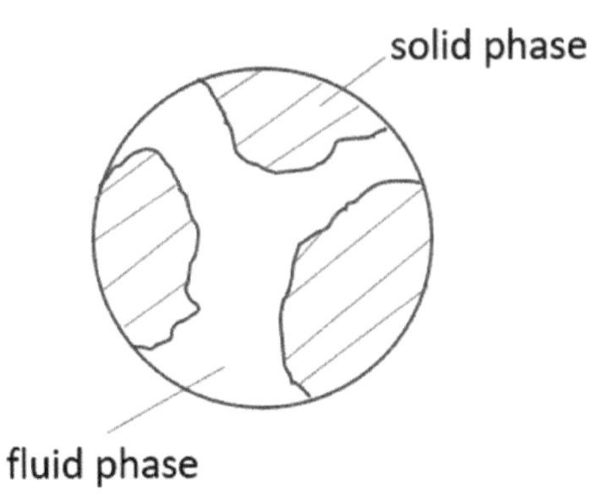

FIGURE 8.1 One material point of porous media.

Substituting Equation (8.2) into the above equation yields:

$$\nabla \cdot \left(-k\nabla p\right) + \alpha \dot{\varepsilon}_V + \frac{\dot{p}}{Q^*} = 0. \quad (8.4)$$

The porous media are discretized with the shape functions for the displacements and pore pressure expressed by:

$$\mathbf{u} = \mathbf{N}_s^{\mathrm{T}} \mathbf{u}_e \quad (8.5)$$

$$p = \mathbf{N}_p^{\mathrm{T}} \mathbf{p}_e \quad (8.6)$$

Similar to Equation (4.7), taking the weak form of the Equations (8.1 and 8.4) and selecting the shape functions as the testing function yield the finite element matrix form of the Equations (8.1 and 8.4) [2,3].

$$\begin{bmatrix} \mathbf{M}^{ss} & 0 \\ 0 & 0 \end{bmatrix} \begin{Bmatrix} \ddot{\mathbf{u}} \\ \ddot{\mathbf{p}} \end{Bmatrix} + \begin{bmatrix} 0 & 0 \\ \mathbf{C}^{ps} & \mathbf{C}^{pp} \end{bmatrix} \begin{Bmatrix} \dot{\mathbf{u}} \\ \dot{\mathbf{p}} \end{Bmatrix} + \begin{bmatrix} \mathbf{K}^{ss} & \mathbf{K}^{sp} \\ 0 & \mathbf{K}^{pp} \end{bmatrix} \begin{Bmatrix} \mathbf{u} \\ \mathbf{p} \end{Bmatrix} = \begin{Bmatrix} \mathbf{f}^s \\ \mathbf{f}_p \end{Bmatrix} \quad (8.7)$$

where:

$$\mathbf{M}^{ss} = \int_\Omega \left(\mathbf{N}_s\right)^{\mathrm{T}} \rho \mathbf{N}_s \mathrm{d}\Omega \quad (8.8)$$

$$\mathbf{K}^{ss} = \int_\Omega \mathbf{B} \cdot \mathbf{D}\mathbf{B} \mathrm{d}\Omega \quad (8.9)$$

$$\mathbf{K}^{sp} = -\int_\Omega \mathbf{B} \cdot \alpha \mathbf{I} \mathbf{N}_p \mathrm{d}\Omega \quad (8.10)$$

$$\mathbf{C}^{ps} = \int_{\Omega} \mathbf{N}_p \cdot \alpha \mathbf{I} \cdot \mathbf{B} d\Omega \tag{8.11}$$

$$\mathbf{C}^{pp} = \int_{\Omega} \mathbf{N}_p \cdot \frac{1}{Q^*} \mathbf{N}_p d\Omega \tag{8.12}$$

$$\mathbf{K}^{pp} = \int_{\Omega} \nabla \mathbf{N}_p \cdot k \nabla \mathbf{N}_p d\Omega \tag{8.13}$$

$$\mathbf{f}^{s} = \int_{\Omega} \mathbf{N}_s \cdot \rho \mathbf{b} d\Omega + \int_{\Gamma} \mathbf{N}_s \cdot \mathbf{t} d\Gamma \tag{8.14}$$

$$\mathbf{f}_p = \int_{\Gamma} \mathbf{N}_p \cdot \mathbf{q} d\Gamma. \tag{8.15}$$

Equations (8.14 and 8.15) are linked with the surface traction **t** and flow flux **q** at the boundary, respectively.

In Equation (8.7), the terms $\mathbf{K}^{sp}$ and $\mathbf{C}^{ps}$ are coupling terms between the solid phase and fluid phase. Equation (8.7) was implemented in ANSYS as coupled pore-pressured-thermal (CPT) elements.

8.2 FINITE ELEMENT PROCEDURE OF POROUS MEDIA IN ANSYS

The following points outline the general procedure to build a finite element model of porous media:

1. *Build the model*: The model can be built in MADPL and ANSYS Workbench.
2. *Set up the model environment*: CPT elements CPT212/213/215/216/217 with u and p as DOFs are available in ANSYS to build the biphasic model. Keyopt(12)=1 should be defined to specify p as one of DOFs.
3. *Define the material properties*: The material properties of porous media, including permeability and Biot coefficient, are defined by TB and PM commands in ANSYS.
4. *Mesh the model*: The meshing of porous media is similar to the structural meshing.
5. *Define the boundary conditions and loadings*: The boundary conditions and loadings are specified in ANSYS using SF, D, and BF commands. For example, the pore pressure at the boundary condition is defined by command D, PRES.
6. *Solve the equation*: The matrix form (Equation [8.7]) is unsymmetrical. Thus, the unsymmetrical option for the Newton-Raphson method should be turned on by the command NROPT, UNSYM.
7. *Post-process the analysis*: After solution, the results, including pore pressure, can be reviewed in both POST1 and POST26 of ANSYS.

8.3 FINITE ELEMENT ANALYSIS OF BIOLOGICAL TISSUE IN THE CONFINED COMPRESSION TEST

Biological tissues such as articular cartilages are composed of a solid matrix phase, an interstitial fluid phase, and an ion phase [4]. The material properties of biological tissues, especially the permeability of the biological tissues, can be measured by the confined compression test. This test is normally performed by confining biological tissues within a cylinder over a porous filter to allow free fluid flow, and applying the loading on the tissue specimen by a nonporous indenter (Figure 8.2) [5]. The creep response of biological tissues in the confined compression test can be used to determine the material properties of biological tissues like Young's modulus and the permeability. To reveal the relation between the creep response of biological tissues and their material properties, this study simulated the creep response of biological tissues in the confined compression test using CPT solid elements.

8.3.1 Finite Element Model

A two-dimensional axisymmetrical model of biological tissue with a radius of 2 mm and height of 10 mm was created to simulate the tissue specimen (Figure 8.3). The model was meshed by using CPT212 with Keyopt(3)=1, which was defined in ANSYS as:

```
ET,1,CPT212              ! COUPLED PORE-PRESSURE-THERMAL (CPT)
KEYOPT,1,3,1             ! AXISYMMETRICAL
KEYOPT,1,12,1
```

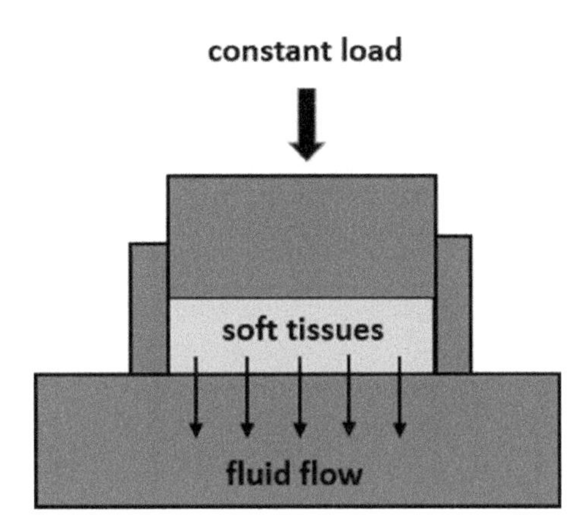

FIGURE 8.2 Schematic of the confined compression test. (From Maas, S.A. et al., *J. Biomech. Eng.*, 34, 011005 (10 pages), 2012.)

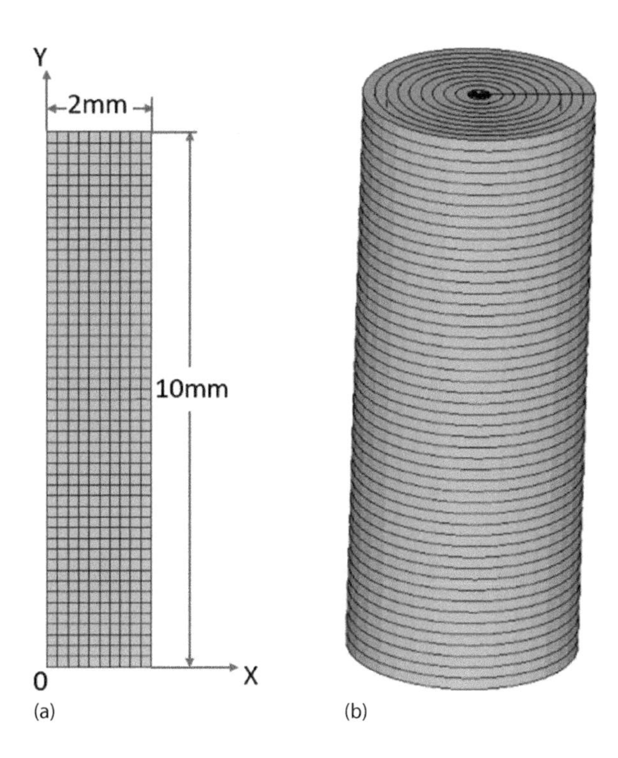

FIGURE 8.3 Finite element model of the soft tissue: (a) two-dimensional axisymmetrical model and (b) three-dimensional model.

8.3.2 Material Properties

The biological tissue was assumed as linear elastic with Young's modulus 15 kPa and Poisson's ratio 0.49. The permeability of the biological tissue was assigned as 8e-2 $mm^4/N \cdot S$ and specified in ANSYS by:

```
FPX=8e-2                    ! mm^4/N.S
ONE=1.0
TB,PM,1,,,PERM              ! Permeability
TBDATA,1,FPX
TB,PM,1,,,BIOT             ! BIOT COEFFICIENT
TBDATA,1,ONE
```

8.3.3 Boundary Conditions and Loadings

The top edge was loaded with pressure 1 kPa, the bottom edge was fixed in the vertical direction, and the right edge was constrained in the axial direction

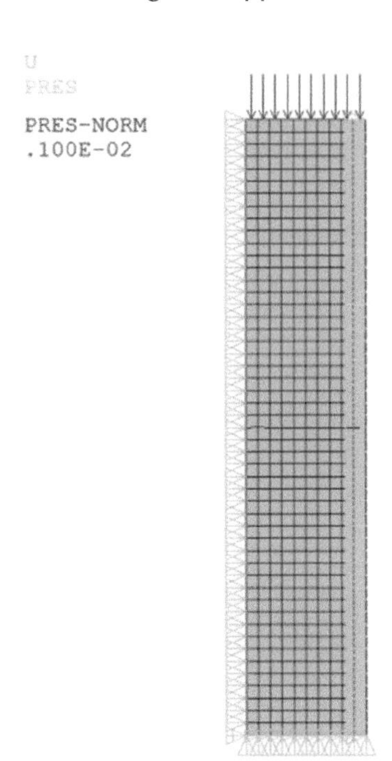

FIGURE 8.4 Boundary conditions and loadings.

because it was a confined compression test (Figure 8.4). Zero pore pressure was given at the bottom to allow the fluid flow:

```
NSEL,S,LOC,Y,0
D,ALL,UY,0
D,ALL,PRES,0
ALLSEL
```

8.3.4 Solution Setting

Large deflection effects were included by command NLGEOM, ON. Stepped loading was specified by command KBC, 1. The whole loading time was 10,000 seconds (about 2.78 hours).

8.3.5 Results

Figure 8.5 plots the results of pore pressure at the end of the first step and the last step. At the end of the first step (Figure 8.5a), most of the pore pressures are close to the loading pressure 1 kPa, except for the part close to the bottom, because zero pore pressure was assigned to the bottom edge in the boundary conditions. In Figure 8.5b, after 10,000 seconds, all pore pressures in the biological tissues are approximately zero.

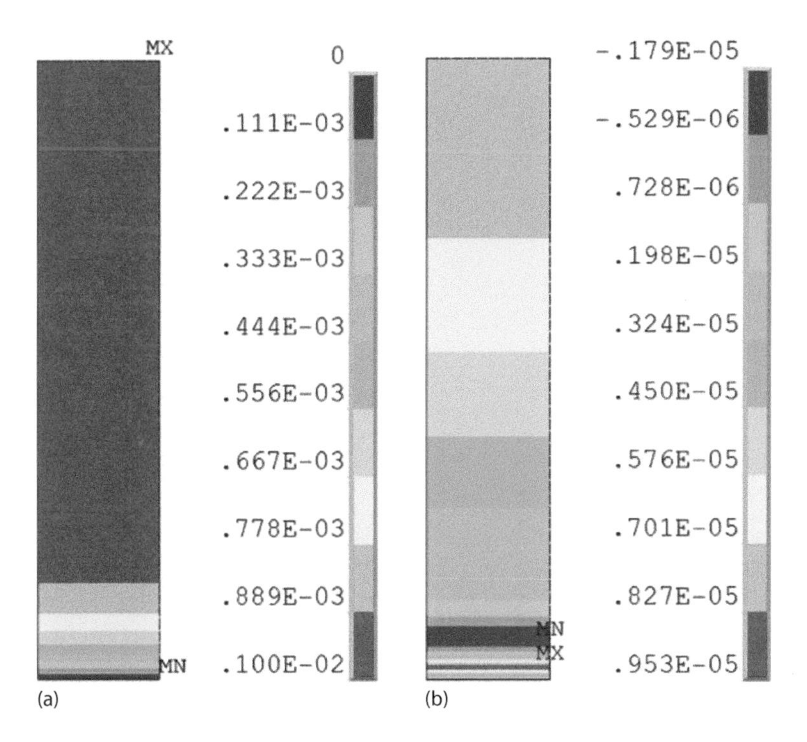

FIGURE 8.5 Pore pressure contour: (a) pore pressures at the end of the first step (MPa) and (b) pore pressures at the end of the last step (MPa).

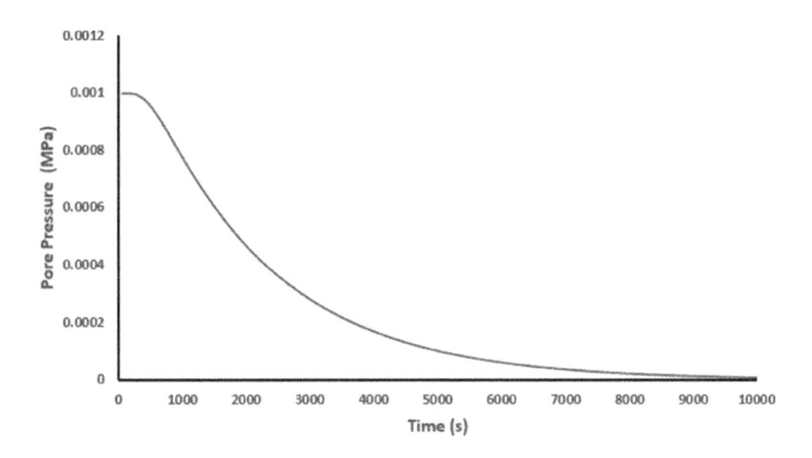

FIGURE 8.6 Time history of pore pressure close to the top edge.

The time history of the pore pressure at the top edge is presented in Figure 8.6. It starts with 1 kPa, decreases gradually, and finally approaches to zero, which is consistent with the results of Figure 8.5. Similarly, the vertical displacement of the top edge drops with time and finally approaches a constant 0.039 mm (Figure 8.7), which matches the reference results well [6].

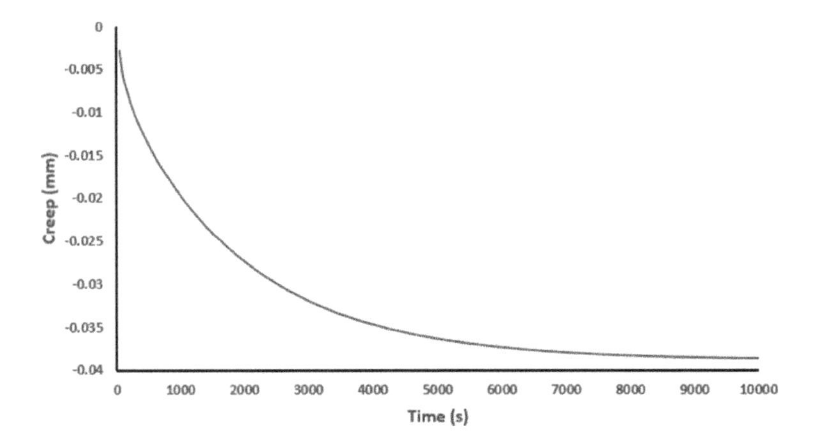

FIGURE 8.7 Time history of vertical displacement of the top edge.

8.3.6 Discussion

A two-dimensional axisymmetrical finite element model with CPT212 was developed to simulate the biological tissues in the confined compression test. The vertical displacement of the top edge decreases with time and approaches to one constant, which matches the references well. Thus, the finite element results verify the creep response of the biological tissues. If the biological tissues are modeled as only elastic, the vertical displacement would keep one constant and not decrease with time. This shows the advantage of modeling biological tissues as porous media with CPT elements.

The biological tissues are biphasic with the solid and fluid phases. The creep response of the biological tissues results from the interaction between the fluid and the solid phases. In addition, the fluid flow in the biological tissues is governed by Darcy's law, which is directly related to the permeability of the fluid. Therefore, the permeability of the biological tissues can be measured from the creep response of the biological tissues.

8.3.7 Summary

The creep response of the biological tissues in the confined compression test was simulated using CPT elements in ANSYS. The computational results match the reference well. The permeability of the biological tissues can be determined from the creep response of the biological tissues.

REFERENCES

1. Inoue, H., "Three-dimensional architecture of lumbar intervertebral disc," *Spine*, Vol. 6, 1981, pp. 139–146.
2. Simon, B.R., Zienkiewicz, O.C., and Paul, D.K., "An analytical solution for the transient response of saturated porous elastic solids," *International Journal for Numerical and Analytical Methods in Geomechanics*, Vol. 8, 1984, pp. 381–398.

3. ANSYS help documentation in the help page of ANSYS190 Product.
4. Lai, W.M., Hou, J.S., and Mow, V.C., "A triphasic theory for the swelling and deformation behavior of articular cartilage," *ASME Journal of Biomechanical Engineering*, Vol. 113, 1991, pp. 245–258.
5. Boschetti, F., Pennati, G., Scienza, F., Gervaso, F., Colombo, M., Peretti, G.M., and Passi, A., "Depth dependent creep response of human articular cartilage during compression: Experimental testing and simulation," *2003 Summer Bioengineering Conference*, June 25–29, Sonesta Beach Resort, Key Biscayne, FL, pp. 1139–1140.
6. Maas, S.A., Ateshian, G.A., and Weiss, J.A., "FEBio: Finite elements for biomechanics," *Journal of Biomechanical Engineering*, Vol. 34, 2012, 011005 (10 pages).

9 Acoustic-Structural Coupling

Acoustic problems are always associated with solid structures. For example, the deformation of the tympanic membrane (TM) is often caused by acoustic pressure in the ear. Thus, these acoustic problems should be modeled by acoustic-structural coupling.

Chapter 9 first presents the governing equations of acoustic-structural coupling and the corresponding finite element modeling procedure in ANSYS. It then shows a simulation of the blast wave transmission through the human ear.

9.1 FINITE ELEMENT MATRIX OF ACOUSTIC-STRUCTURAL COUPLING

At the acoustic fluid-structure interaction (FSI), integrating pressure over the area of the interface (Figure 9.1b), the acoustic pressure load vector can be expressed as [1]:

$$\mathbf{f}_e^{pr} = \mathbf{R}_e \mathbf{p}_e \tag{9.1}$$

where:

$\mathbf{R}_e$—transformation matrix from $\mathbf{p}_e$ to $\mathbf{f}_e^{pr}$.

$$\mathbf{R}_e = \int_{\Gamma_0} \mathbf{N}_s \mathbf{n} \mathbf{N}_p^{\mathrm{T}} d\Gamma \tag{9.2}$$

where:

$\mathbf{N}_s$ = shape function of displacement in structure element;
$\mathbf{N}_p$ = shape function of acoustic pressure in acoustic fluid element; and
$\mathbf{n}$ = unit normal on the coupling interface of the fluid element.

Thus, the equilibrium equation of the structural element (2.12) with the additional external force from the acoustic domain $\mathbf{f}_e^{pr}$ is written as:

$$\mathbf{M}_e^s \ddot{\mathbf{u}}_e + \mathbf{C}_e^s \dot{\mathbf{u}}_e + \mathbf{K}_e^s \mathbf{u}_e = \mathbf{f}_e^s + \mathbf{f}_e^{pr} \tag{9.3}$$

Substituting Equation (9.1) into the above equation yields:

$$\mathbf{M}_e^s \ddot{\mathbf{u}}_e + \mathbf{C}_e^s \dot{\mathbf{u}}_e + \mathbf{K}_e^s \mathbf{u}_e - \mathbf{R}_e \mathbf{p}_e = \mathbf{f}_e^s \tag{9.4}$$

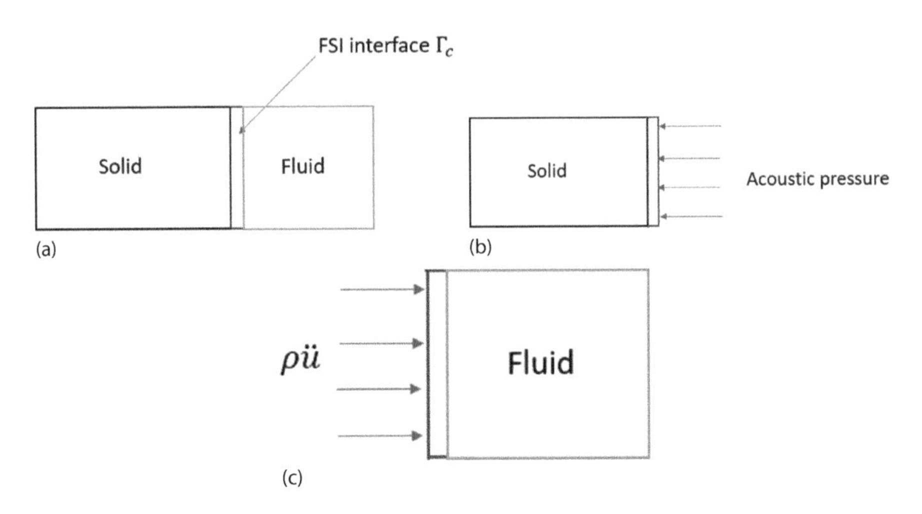

FIGURE 9.1 Acoustic-structural coupling: (a) acoustic FSI, (b) structural part of FSI, and (c) fluid part of FSI.

When acoustic FSI exists, Equation (4.7) becomes:

$$\int_{\Omega_f} \frac{1}{c^2} \delta p \frac{\partial^2 p}{\partial t^2} \mathrm{d}\Omega + \int_{\Omega_f} \frac{\partial(\delta p)}{\partial x_i} \frac{\partial p}{\partial x_i} \mathrm{d}\Omega + \int_{\Gamma_0} \delta p \left[\frac{r}{\rho_0 c} \right] \frac{1}{c} \frac{\partial p}{\partial t} \mathrm{d}\Gamma = \int_{\Gamma_0} n_i \delta p \frac{\partial p}{\partial x_i} \mathrm{d}\Gamma \tag{9.5}$$

The right term takes the acoustic pressure at the boundary into account (Figure 9.1).

In acoustic-structural coupling, the normal pressure gradient of the fluid and the normal acceleration of the structure results in the following relation [1]:

$$n_i \frac{\partial p}{\partial x_i} = -\rho_0 n_i \frac{\partial^2 u_i}{\partial t^2} \tag{9.6}$$

After discretization, the acceleration of the structure is expressed in terms of shape function and element nodal displacement,

$$\frac{\partial^2 \boldsymbol{u}}{\partial t^2} = \mathbf{N}_s^{\mathrm{T}} \ddot{\mathbf{u}}_e \tag{9.7}$$

Substituting Equations (9.6 and 9.7) into Equation (9.5) yields the matrix form of the acoustic governing equation:

$$\mathbf{M}_e^p \ddot{\mathbf{p}}_e + \mathbf{C}_e^p \dot{\mathbf{p}}_e + \mathbf{K}_e^p \mathbf{p}_e + \rho_0 \mathbf{R}_e^{\mathrm{T}} \ddot{\mathbf{u}}_e = 0 \tag{9.8}$$

Compared to Equation (4.12), the above equation has one extra term $\rho_0 \mathbf{R}_e^{\mathrm{T}} \ddot{\mathbf{u}}_e$ to indicate the acoustic-structural interaction.

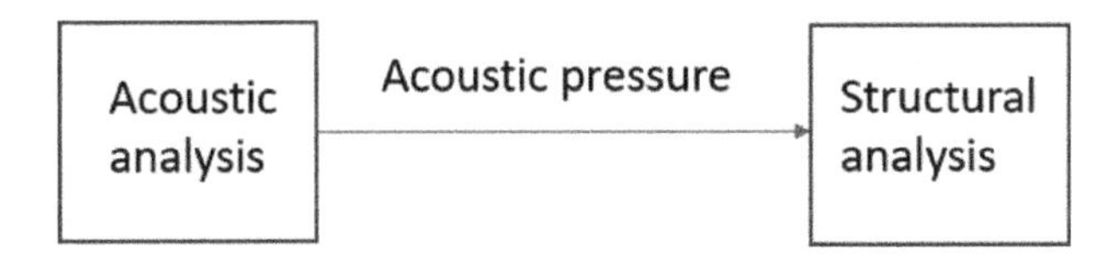

FIGURE 9.2 One-way coupling of acoustic FSI.

Combining Equations (9.4 and 9.8) has the following matrix form [1]:

$$\begin{bmatrix} \mathbf{M}_e^s & 0 \\ \rho_0 \mathbf{R}_e^{\mathrm{T}} & \mathbf{M}_e^p \end{bmatrix} \begin{Bmatrix} \ddot{\mathbf{u}}_e \\ \ddot{\mathbf{p}}_e \end{Bmatrix} + \begin{bmatrix} \mathbf{C}_e^s & 0 \\ 0 & \mathbf{C}_e^p \end{bmatrix} \begin{Bmatrix} \dot{\mathbf{u}}_e \\ \dot{\mathbf{p}}_e \end{Bmatrix} + \begin{bmatrix} \mathbf{K}_e^s & -\mathbf{R}_e \\ 0 & \mathbf{K}_e^p \end{bmatrix} \begin{Bmatrix} \mathbf{u}_e \\ \mathbf{p}_e \end{Bmatrix} = \begin{Bmatrix} \mathbf{f}_e^s \\ 0 \end{Bmatrix} \tag{9.9}$$

Equation (9.9) can be directly solved by the sparse solver with acoustic pressure and displacement updated at the same time. Moreover, since the acoustic pressure is very low and causes an extremely small displacement of the solid, this coupling equation can also be solved in a weak manner, in which the acoustic problem is first solved; next, the acoustic pressures are transferred to the solid part, then the structural analysis is performed (Figure 9.2).

Equation (9.9) was implemented in ANSYS as acoustic FSI, which is Keyopt(2)=0 of the acoustic elements.

9.2 FINITE ELEMENT PROCEDURE OF ACOUSTIC FSI IN ANSYS

The following outlines the general procedure to build an acoustic FSI finite element model:

1. *Build the model*: An acoustic FSI model consists of a fluid domain, structural components, FSI interfaces, and the truncation of the infinite domain if the infinite domain exists. The model can be built in the ANSYS Workbench.
2. *Set up the model environment*: Acoustic elements FLUID29, FLUID30, FLUID220, and FLUID221 are available in ANSYS to build the acoustic model. These elements present coupling and no coupling with Keyopt(2)=0 and 1, respectively.
   The solid elements such as PLANE182/183 and SOLID185/186/187 can be used for the structural model.
3. *Define the material properties*: The acoustic material properties, such as density and sonic velocity, and the structural material properties, like Young's modulus and Poisson's ratio, can be defined by MP or TB commands in ANSYS.

4. *Mesh the model*: The structural meshing and acoustic meshing follow the individual requirements, which are specified in Chapters 2 and 4, respectively.
5. *Define the boundary conditions and loadings*: The boundary conditions and loadings are defined in ANSYS using SF, D, and BF commands.
6. *FSI definition*: Command SF,,FSI is used to define a fluid-structure interaction flag in the model.
7. *Solve the equation*: The FSI matrix, Equation (9.9), is unsymmetrical. Thus, it requires a corresponding unsymmetric eigensolver.
8. *Post-process the analysis*: Like in Chapters 2 and 4, the acoustic and structural results can be reviewed in both POST1 and POST26 of ANSYS after solution.

9.3 FINITE ELEMENT ANALYSIS OF BLAST WAVE TRANSMISSION THROUGH HUMAN EAR

More than 60% of injured military members have TM injuries, tinnitus, and hearing loss [2,3], which are primarily caused by the blast wave on the TM and middle ear. Therefore, TM injuries have been studied extensively in animals and humans [4–7]. This study simulated the blast wave transmission through the ear in ANSYS190.

9.3.1 Finite Element Model

The human ear was simplified to comprise the ear canal, TM, and middle ear (ME) cavity (Figure 9.3) [6]. The canal was modeled as a tapered cylinder with length 30 mm; the diameter decreased from 12 mm at the canal entrance to 8 mm near the TM. The TM separated the ear canal and ME cavity.

The TM was modeled by SOLID187 in ANSYS. The ear canal and ME cavity were meshed by FLUID221 (Figure 9.4). The elements between the solid elements and fluid elements were specified as acoustic FSI by FLUID221 with Keyopt(2)=0 (Figure 9.4), which was completed automatically by the program.

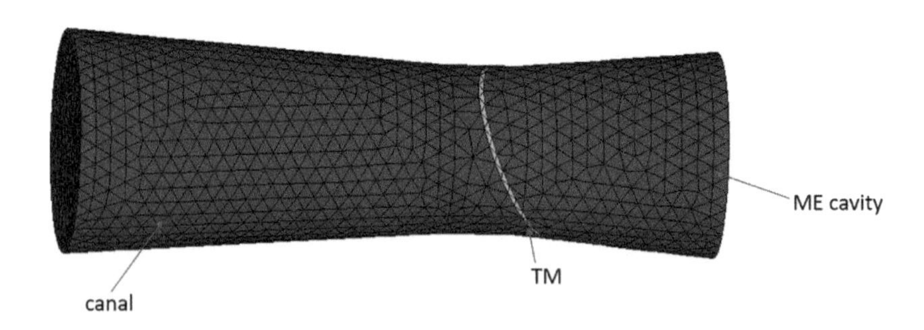

FIGURE 9.3 Finite element model of an ear.

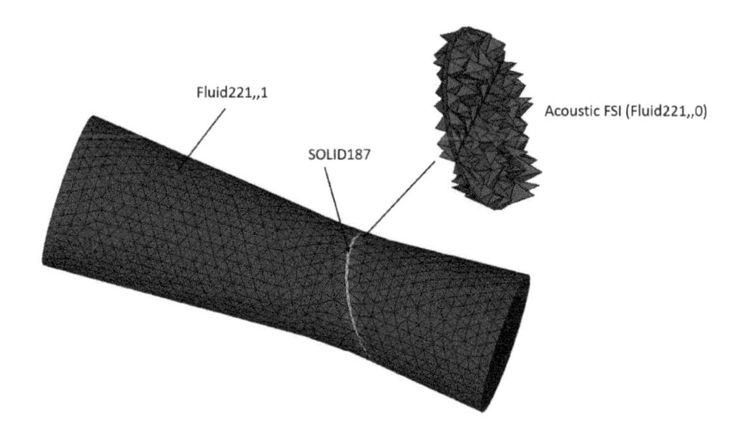

FIGURE 9.4 Various element types in the acoustic finite element model.

9.3.2 Material Properties

The TM was assumed to be viscoelastic and modeled by the Prony series in ANSYS.

```
ALPHA=0.66
TAU=25E-6
MP,EX,1,23E6                                    ! PA
MP,NUXY,1,0.3
MP,DENS,1,1200                                  ! KG/M^3
TB,PRONY,1,,1,SHEAR
TBDATA,1,ALPHA,TAU

TB,PRONY,1,,1,BULK
TBDATA,1,ALPHA,TAU
```

The ear canal and ME cavity were assigned acoustic material properties.

```
MP,DENS,2,1.21                                  ! DENSITY
MP,SONC,2,343                                   ! SONIC VELOCITY
```

9.3.3 Loadings and Boundary Conditions

The entrance of the ear canal was loaded with a blast presented by the time history of acoustic pressure (Figure 9.5), which was defined in ANSYS as:

```
*DIM,_LOADVARI,TABLE,3,1,1,TIME,
! TIME VALUES
_LOADVARI(1,0,1) = 0.
_LOADVARI(2,0,1) = 0.5E-3
_LOADVARI(3,0,1) = 2E-3

! LOAD VALUES
_LOADVARI(1,1,1) = 1E4.
```

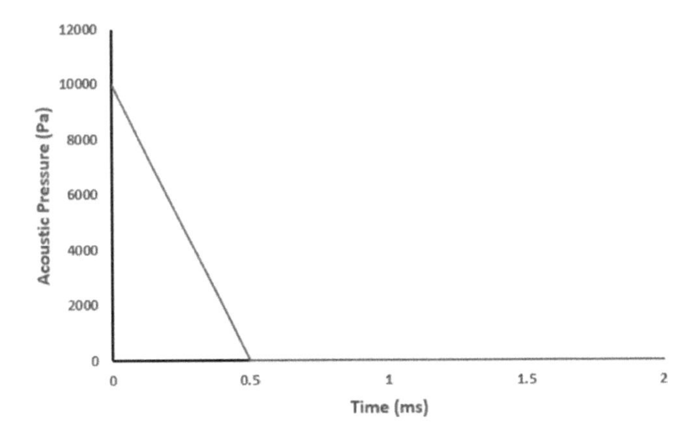

FIGURE 9.5 Time history of a blast.

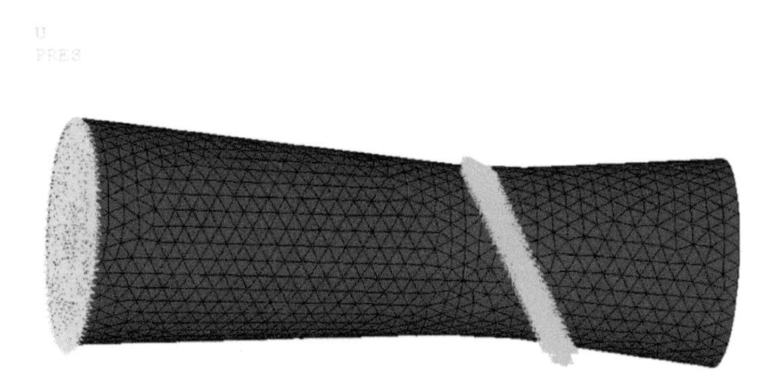

FIGURE 9.6 Boundary conditions.

```
_LOADVARI(2,1,1) = 0
_LOADVARI(3,1,1) = 0

ASEL,S,AREA,,1
NSLA,S,1
D,ALL,PRES,%_LOADVARI%
ALLSEL
```

The TM was constrained at the boundary with all degrees of freedom (Figure 9.6).

9.3.4 Solution Setting

A transient analysis was conducted to simulate the response of the human ear in 2 ms after the blast. A stepped loading option was turned on by KBC,1.

9.3.5 Results

Figure 9.7 presents the acoustic pressures of the human ear from 0.024 to 2 ms, which indicates that the acoustic wave transits gradually from the entrance of the ear canal to the TM at time 0.1 ms, then through TM to the ME cavity. The time history of the acoustic pressures of points P0, P1, and P2 is shown in Figure 9.8. Figure 9.8b is very close to reference [6]. The P0 in Figure 9.8c matches the loading history of Figure 9.5. The results of P1 show that the acoustic pressure decays gradually. The results of P2

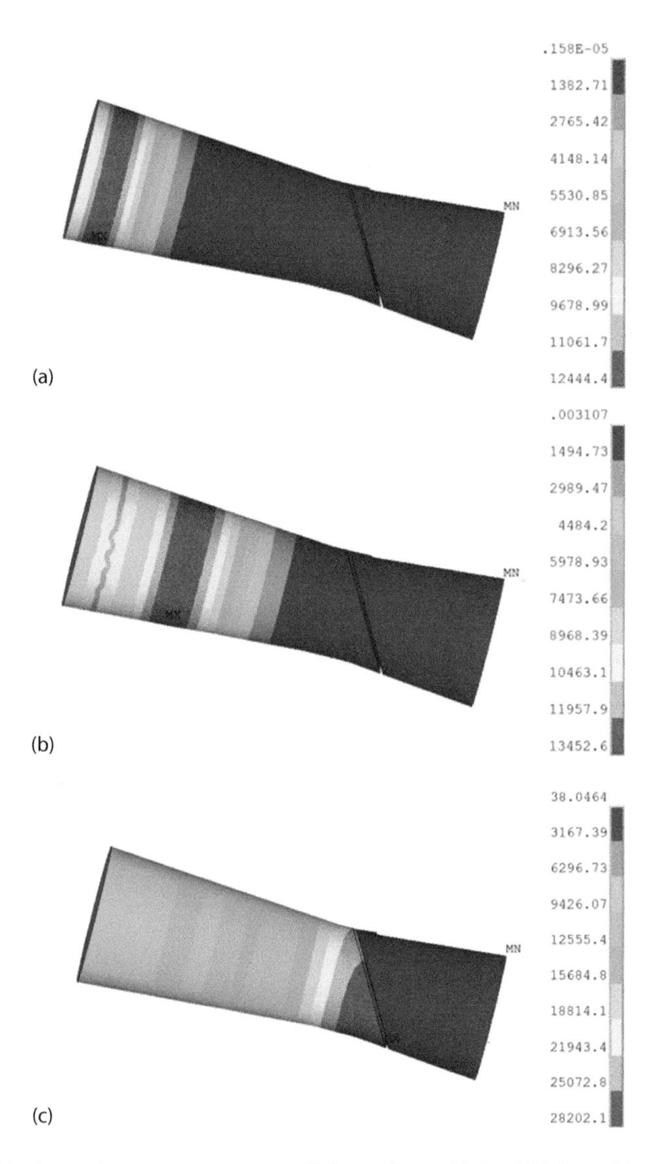

FIGURE 9.7 Acoustic pressure contour at different times: (a) $T = 0.024$ ms, (b) $T = 0.048$ ms, (c) $T = 0.1$ ms. *(Continued)*

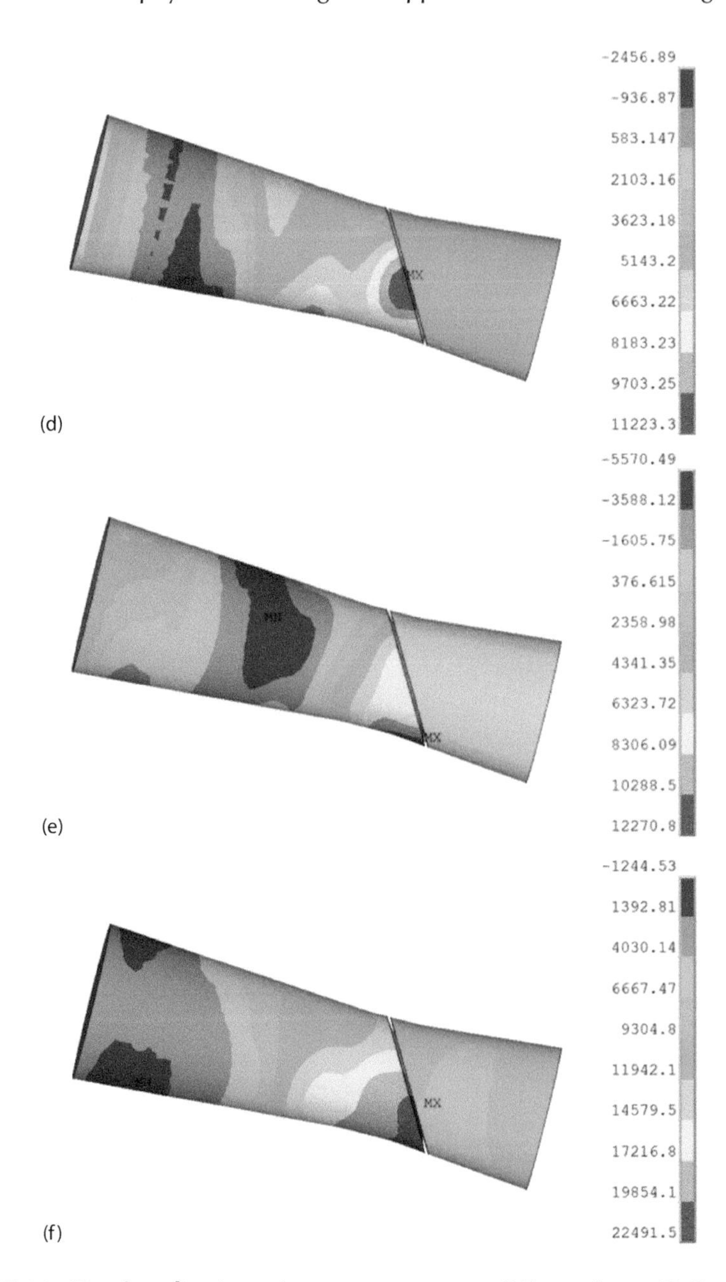

FIGURE 9.7 (Continued) Acoustic pressure contour at different times: (d) T = 0.2 ms, (e) T = 0.3 ms, (f) T = 0.4 ms. *(Continued)*

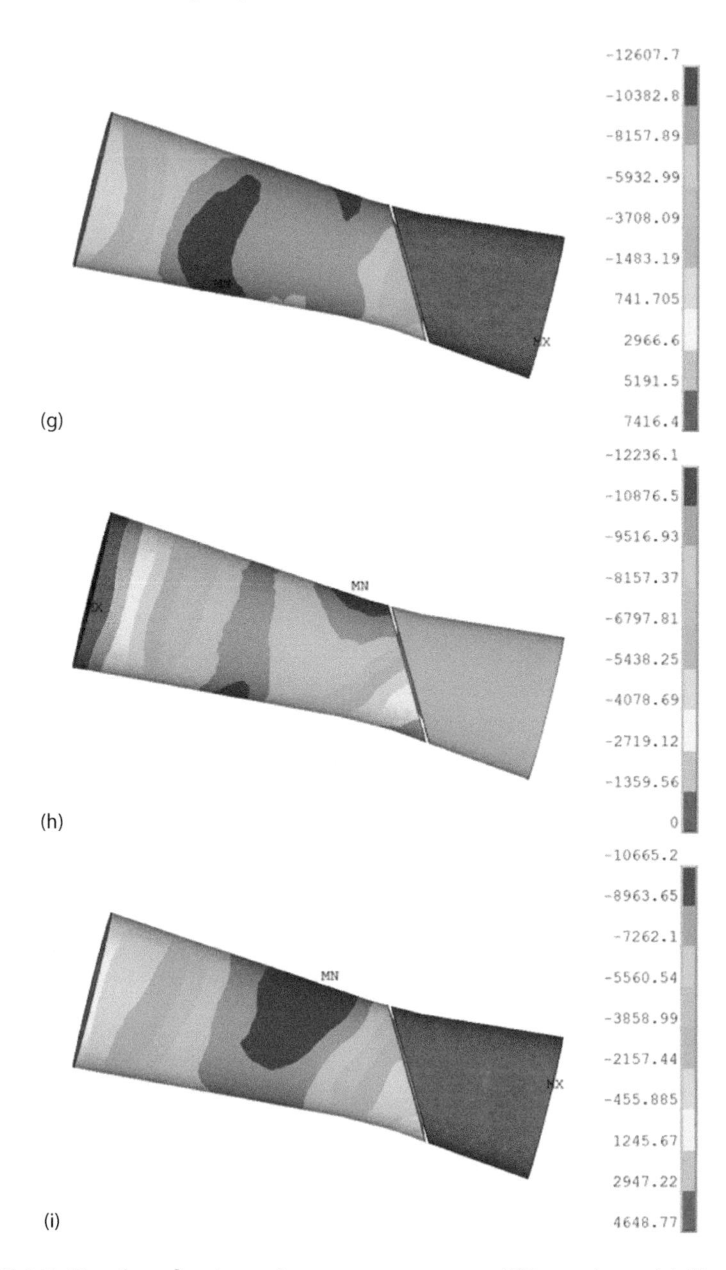

FIGURE 9.7 (Continued) Acoustic pressure contour at different times: (g) $T = 0.5$ ms, (h) $T = 1.0$ ms, (i) $T = 1.5$ ms. *(Continued)*

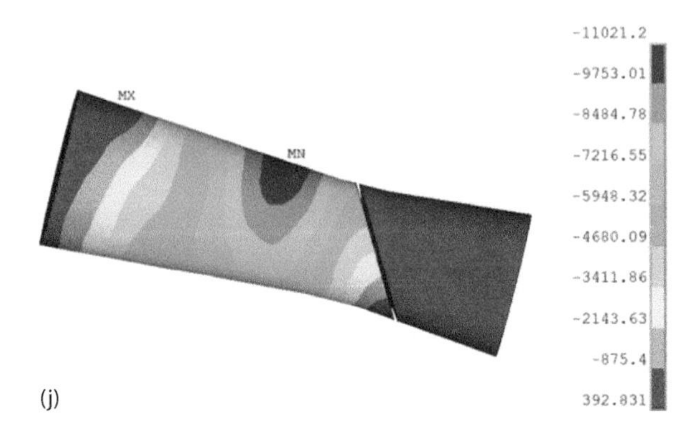

FIGURE 9.7 (Continued) Acoustic pressure contour at different times: (j) $T = 2$ ms.

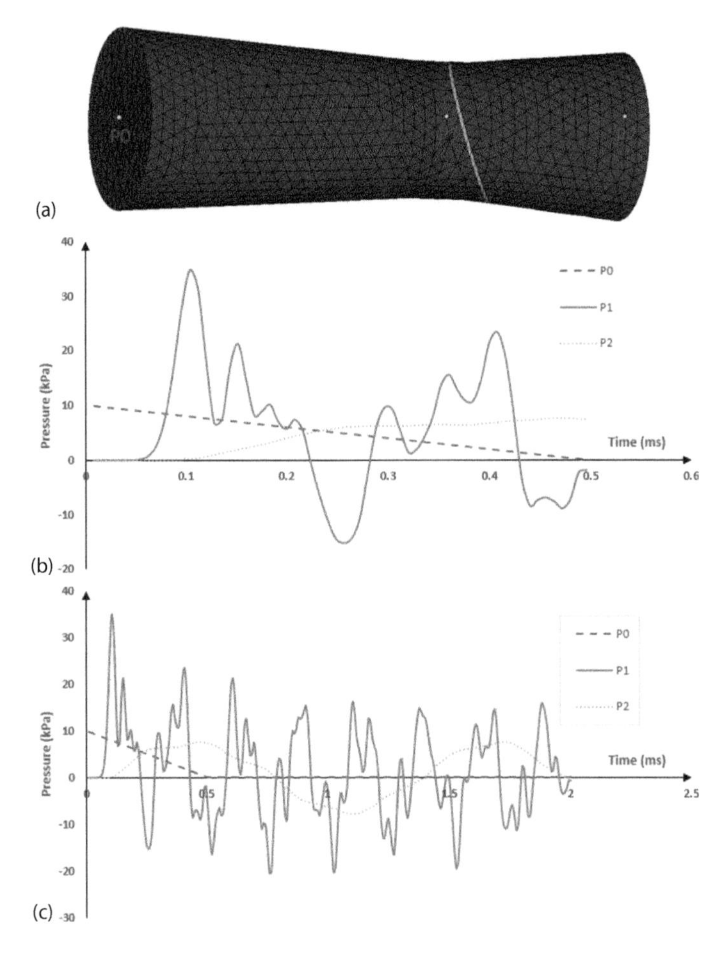

FIGURE 9.8 Time history of acoustic pressures of P0, P1, and P2: (a) locations of P0, P1, and P2, (b) time history in 0.5 ms, and (c) time history in 2 ms.

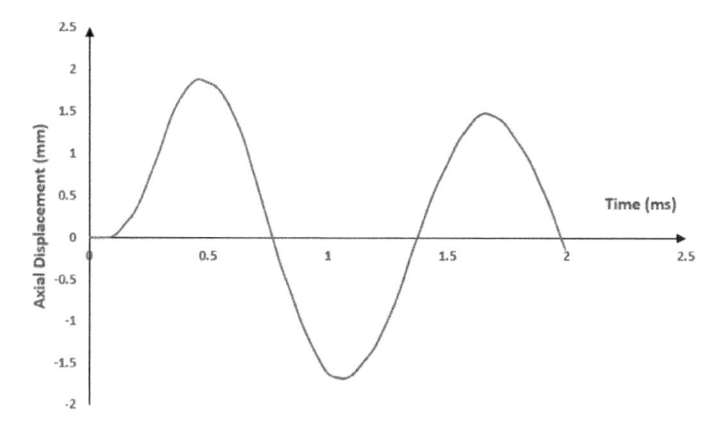

FIGURE 9.9 Axial displacement of TM with time.

are close to those of the axial displacement of the TM (Figure 9.9), which suggests the connection of the acoustic wave in the ME cavity with the vibration of the TM.

The deformation and vM stresses of the TM at time 0.5 ms, with the maximum deformation 2.1 mm and maximum stress 0.69 MPa, are plotted in Figure 9.10.

9.3.6 Discussion

A finite element model of a human ear was built to simulate the blast wave transmission through the ear. The time history of acoustic pressures in the ear canal and ME cavity was presented, and the deformation and stresses of the TM were obtained, which can be applied for further research of the TM injuries.

The whole finite element model consisted of the solid part (TM), the acoustic part (ear canal and ME cavity), and the acoustic FSI. Therefore, the TM was meshed by SOLID187, the ear canal and ME cavity were meshed by FLUID221 with Keyopt(2)=1, and the FSI part was meshed by FLUID221 with Keyopt(2)=0. Different element types correspond to the different governing equations.

9.3.7 Summary

A blast wave transmission through the human ear was simulated in ANSYS190. The deformations and stresses of the TM were obtained for further study of TM.

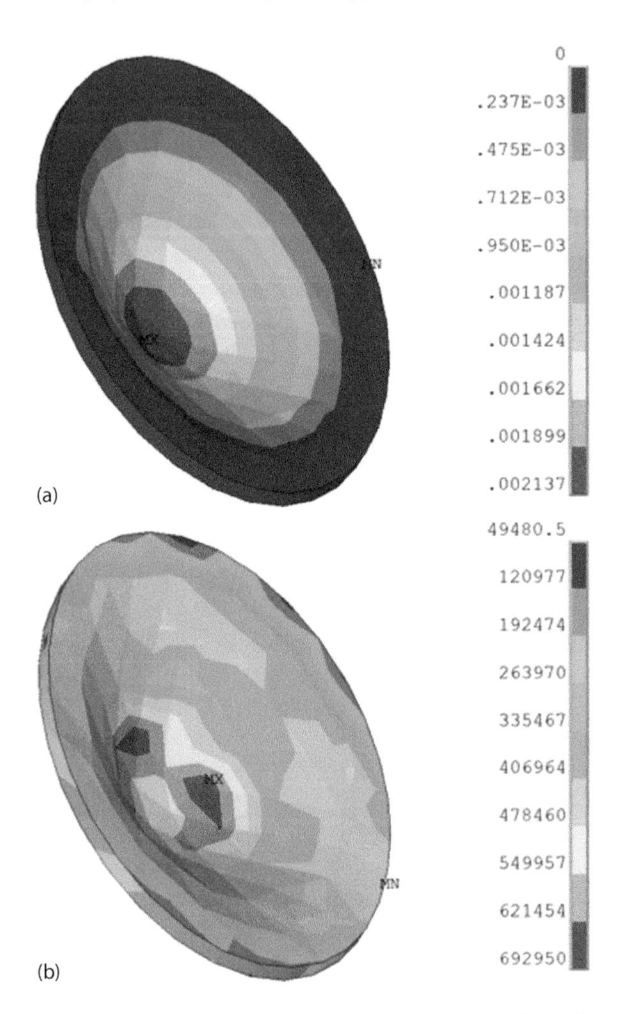

FIGURE 9.10 Deformation and stresses of TM at t = 0.5 ms: (a) deformation (m) and (b) vM stresses (Pa).

REFERENCES

1. Zhang, Q., and Cen, S., *Multiphysics Modeling: Numerical Methods and Engineering Applications*, Academic Press, Cambridge, MA, January 2016.
2. Helfer, T.M., Jordan, N.N., and Lee, R.B., "Post deployment hearing loss in US Army soldiers seen at audiology clinics from April 1, 2003, through March 31, 2004," *American Journal of Audiology*, Vol. 14, 2005, pp. 161–168.
3. Cave, K.M., Cornish, E.M., and Chandler, D.W., "Blast injury of the ear: Clinical update from the global war on terror," *Journal of Military Medicine*, Vol. 172, 2007, pp. 726–730.
4. Cho, S.I., Gao, S.S., Xia, A., et al., "Mechanisms of hearing loss after blast injury to the ear," *PLOS One*, Vol. 8, 2013, pp. e67618.

5. Fausti, S.A., Wilmington, D.J., Gallun, F.J., Myers, P.J., and Henry, J.A., "Auditory and vestibular dysfunction associated with blast-related traumatic brain injury," *Journal of Rehabilitation Research & Development*, Vol. 46, 2009, pp. 797–810.
6. Leckness, K., *Novel Finite Element Method to Predict Blast Wave Transmission Through Human Ear*, Master Thesis, University of Oklahoma, 2016.
7. Gan, R.Z., Leckness, K., Nakmali, D., and Ji, X.D., "Biomechanical measurement and modeling of human eardrum injury in relation to blast wave direction," *Military Medicine*, Vol. 183, Supplement, 2018, pp. 245–251.

10 Thermal-Structural Coupling

Thermal-structural coupling such as people becoming warm after exercise occurs in the human body. Thus, Chapter 10 discusses thermal-structural coupling, including its governing equation, finite element implementation, and modeling procedure in ANSYS, and presents an application for the study of heat generation of biological tissues under cyclic loading.

10.1 THERMAL-STRESS COUPLING

The stress-strain relation in the coupled thermo-elastic constitutive equations is [1]:

$$\varepsilon = \left[\mathbf{C}\right]^{-1} \sigma + \alpha \Delta T \tag{10.1}$$

where:

$\varepsilon = \left[\varepsilon_x, \varepsilon_y, \varepsilon_z, \varepsilon_{xy}, \varepsilon_{yz}, \varepsilon_{xz}\right]^{\mathrm{T}}$

$\sigma = \left[\sigma_x, \sigma_y, \sigma_z, \sigma_{xy}, \sigma_{yz}, \sigma_{xz}\right]^{\mathrm{T}}$

$\left[\mathbf{C}\right]$ = elastic stiffness matrix

α = vector of coefficients of thermal expansion $= \left[\alpha_x, \alpha_y, \alpha_z, 0, 0, 0\right]^{\mathrm{T}}$.

$$\Delta T = T - T_0 \tag{10.2}$$

T = current temperature

T_0 = reference temperature

To take the thermal strain into account, the equilibrium Equation (2.16) adding the thermal components becomes [2]:

$$\mathbf{M}^s \ddot{\mathbf{u}} + \mathbf{K}^s \mathbf{u} + \mathbf{K}^{sT} \Delta \mathbf{T} = \mathbf{f}^s \tag{10.3}$$

or

$$\mathbf{M}^s \ddot{\mathbf{u}} + \mathbf{K}^s \mathbf{u} + \mathbf{K}^{sT} \mathbf{T} = \mathbf{f}^s + \mathbf{K}^{sT} \mathbf{T}_0 \tag{10.4}$$

where:

$$\mathbf{K}^{sT} = \sum_{e=1}^{ne} \mathbf{K}_e^{sT} \tag{10.5}$$

$$\mathbf{K}_e^{sT} = -\int_{\Omega_e} \mathbf{B}^{\mathrm{T}}\boldsymbol{\beta}\mathbf{N}^{\mathrm{T}} d\Omega \tag{10.6}$$

$$\boldsymbol{\beta} = \mathbf{C}\boldsymbol{\alpha} \tag{10.7}$$

In the case of the material deformation, the heat conductivity Equation (5.1) becomes [2]:

$$\rho c_v \frac{\partial T}{\partial t} = \nabla^{\mathrm{T}}\mathbf{k}\nabla T - T_0\boldsymbol{\beta}^{\mathrm{T}}\frac{\partial \boldsymbol{\varepsilon}}{\partial t} + \rho r \tag{10.8}$$

where:

c_v = specific heat
ρ = mass density
$\mathbf{k}$ = matrix of thermal conductivity
r = energy supply at the element per unit mass

The corresponding matrix form (Equation [5.22]) changes to [2]:

$$\mathbf{C}^T\dot{\mathbf{T}} + \mathbf{K}^{TT}\mathbf{T} + \mathbf{C}^{Ts}\dot{\mathbf{u}} = \mathbf{Q}^T \tag{10.9}$$

where:

$$\mathbf{C}^{Ts} = \sum \mathbf{C}_e^{Ts} \tag{10.10}$$

$$\mathbf{C}_e^{Ts} = T_0\int_{\Omega_e} \mathbf{B}^{\mathrm{T}}\boldsymbol{\beta}\mathbf{N}^{\mathrm{T}} d\Omega \tag{10.11}$$

Therefore, combining Equations (10.4 and 10.9), the thermal-structural-coupled equations have the following form [2]:

$$\begin{bmatrix} \mathbf{M}^s & 0 \\ 0 & 0 \end{bmatrix}\begin{Bmatrix} \ddot{\mathbf{u}} \\ \ddot{\mathbf{T}} \end{Bmatrix} + \begin{bmatrix} 0 & 0 \\ \mathbf{C}^{Ts} & \mathbf{C}^T \end{bmatrix}\begin{Bmatrix} \dot{\mathbf{u}} \\ \dot{\mathbf{T}} \end{Bmatrix} + \begin{bmatrix} \mathbf{K}^s & \mathbf{K}^{sT} \\ 0 & \mathbf{K}^{TT} \end{bmatrix}\begin{Bmatrix} \mathbf{u} \\ \mathbf{T} \end{Bmatrix} = \begin{Bmatrix} \mathbf{f}^s + \mathbf{K}^{sT}\mathbf{T}_0 \\ \mathbf{Q}^T \end{Bmatrix} \tag{10.12}$$

where $\mathbf{C}^{Ts}$ and $\mathbf{K}^{sT}$ are the coupling terms in the above equation.

Equation (10.12) was implemented in ANSYS as a new feature of coupled elements 22x with Keyopt(1)=11.

10.2 FINITE ELEMENT PROCEDURE OF THERMAL-STRUCTURAL ANALYSIS IN ANSYS

The following points outline the general procedure to build a thermal-structural finite element model:

1. *Build the model*: The structural model and thermal model can be different. The data exchange between them must go through mapping. When the structural model is identical to the thermal model, Equation (10.7) can be solved simultaneously with both u and T as degree of freedoms (DOFs).
2. *Set up the model environment*: With both u and T as DOFs, two-dimensional thermal-structural elements PLANE222/223 and three-dimensional thermal-structural elements SOLID226/227 with Keyopt(1)=11 are available for the thermal-structural analysis.
3. *Define the material properties*: The structural material properties, like Young's modulus and Poisson's ratio, and thermal material properties, such as conductivity and specific heat, as well as coupling coefficient QRATE, can be defined by MP or TB commands in ANSYS.
4. *Mesh the model*: The general requirement for meshing is fine with the regular shape.
5. *Define the loadings and boundary conditions*: The loadings and boundary conditions are specified in ANSYS using SF, D, and F commands.
6. *Solve the equation*: The unsymmetrical thermal-structural coupling matrix (Equation [10.12]) requires an unsymmetric eigensolver.
7. *Post-process the analysis*: After solution, the thermal and structural results can be reviewed in both POST1 and POST26 of ANSYS following the approaches in Chapters 2 and 5.

10.3 SIMULATION OF HEATING GENERATION OF BIOLOGICAL TISSUES UNDER CYCLIC LOADING

Biological tissues, such as ligaments and tendons, are regarded as viscoelastic and consist of both elastic and viscoelastic parts (Figure 10.1). Under cyclic loadings, the energy dissipation caused by the viscoelastic part is converted into thermal energy to generate heat. This study simulated heat generation of biological tissues under cyclic loading in ANSYS190 to reveal the relation between the temperature increase and cyclic loading.

10.3.1 Finite Element Model

A two-dimensional axisymmetrical model with a length of 8.51 mm and a radius of 0.73 mm was made to simulate the biological tissue (Figure 10.2) [3]. It was meshed by a coupled-field solid PLANE223 [1], which was defined in ANSYS by commands:

```
ET, 1, 223, 11          ! STRUCTURAL-THERMAL ANALYSIS
KEYOPT, 1, 9, 1
KEYOPT, 1, 3, 1         ! AXISYMMETRICAL OPTION
```

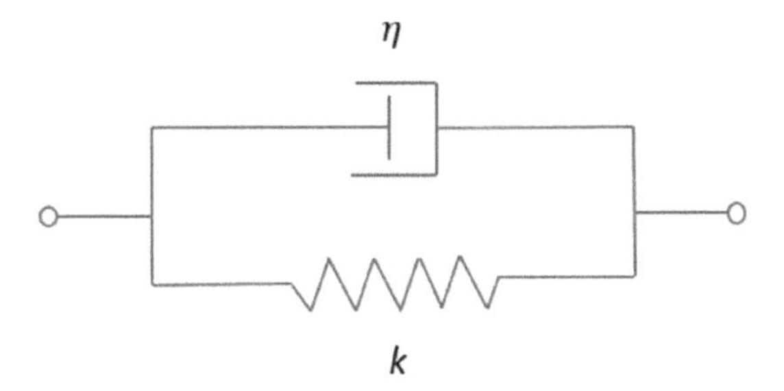

FIGURE 10.1 Schematic of the viscoelastic model.

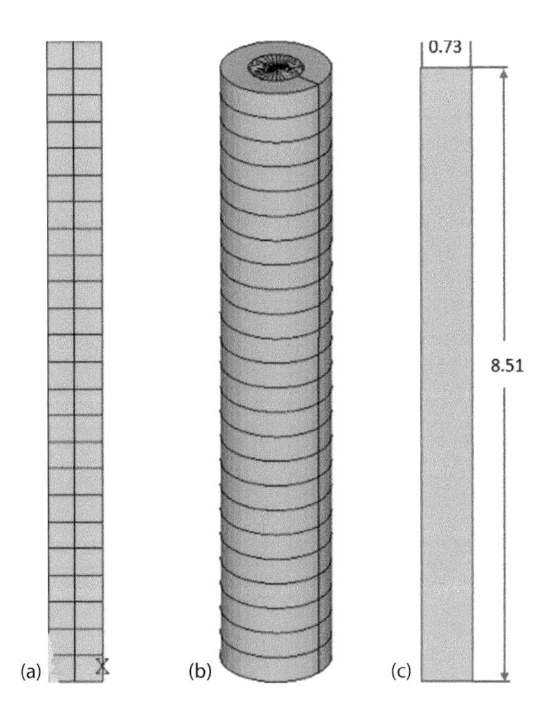

FIGURE 10.2 Finite element model of the soft tissues: (a) 2D axisymmetrical model, (b) 3D model, and (c) dimensions (all dimensions in mm).

10.3.2 Material Properties

The Bergstrom-Boyce model can be applied for the simulation of biological tissues [4]. Thus, the biological tissue was modeled by the Bergstrom-Boyce model with the material parameters listed in Table 10.1.

The analysis also involves thermal analysis. The thermal parameters of the biological tissue are specified in Table 10.2.

TABLE 10.1
Material Parameters of Bergstrom-Boyce Model to Model the Biological Tissue

μ_0(MPa)	N_0	μ_1(MPa)	N_1	$\dot{\gamma}_0 / \tau_{base}^m$	C	m
100	6.86	100	6.86	0.18	−0.16	1.79

TABLE 10.2
Thermal Parameters of the Biological Tissue

Density (kg/mm^3)	Thermal Conductivity (mW/mm K)	Specific Heat (mJ/kg K)	Heat Generation Rate
1.670e-6	0.42	3,000e3	0.9

10.3.3 Boundary Conditions and Loadings

The bottom of the biological tissue was fixed and the top was loaded with cyclic loading (Figure 10.3), which increases linearly with the cyclic numbers (Figure 10.4). The cyclic loading was implemented in ANSYS190 using the following commands:

```
*DO, I, 1, 10
  TIME, (I-1)*10 + 5
  NSEL, S, LOC, Y, LY
  SF, ALL, PRES, -I
  ALLSEL
  SOLVE
  TIME, (I - 1)*10 + 10
  NSEL, S, LOC, Y, LY
  SF, ALL, PRES, 0
  ALLSEL
  SOLVE
*ENDDO
```

The initial temperature was assigned as 36°C.

10.3.4 Solution Setting

A transient analysis was specified with command ANTYPE, TRANS; in addition, large deflection effects were turned on due to the requirement of the Bergstrom-Boyce model.

10.3.5 Results

Figure 10.5 illustrates the whole temperature distribution of the biological tissue after ten cyclic loadings. The temperature is uniformly distributed with 36.0054°C, which indicates that the temperature increases 0.0054°C after ten

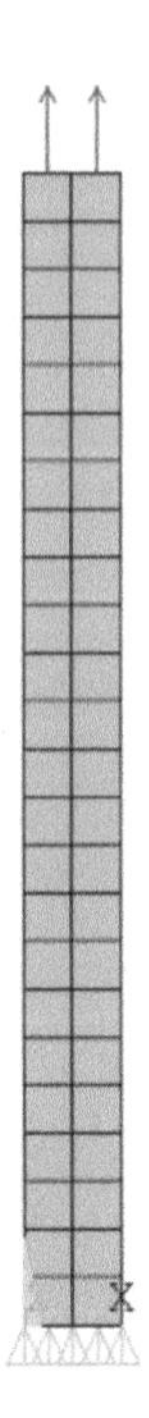

FIGURE 10.3 Boundary conditions.

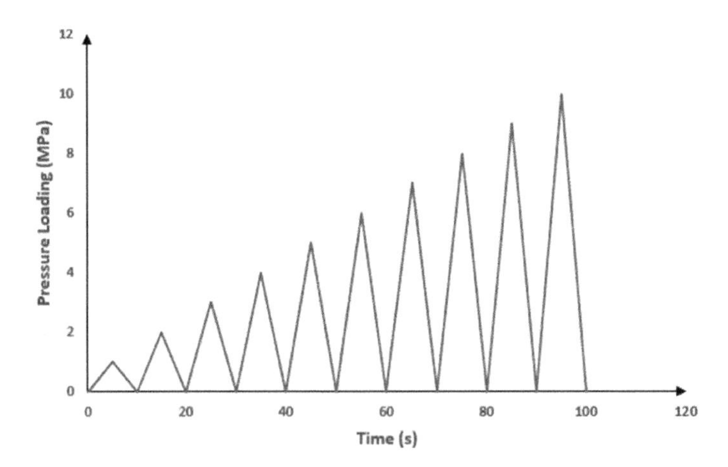

FIGURE 10.4 Variation of tension loading with time.

cyclic loadings. The temperature change with time is presented in Figure 10.6, which shows that the temperature increases with the cyclic loading nonlinearly because the loading increases linearly with the cyclic numbers. Therefore, more mechanical energy is converted into thermal energy to make the temperature increase nonlinearly.

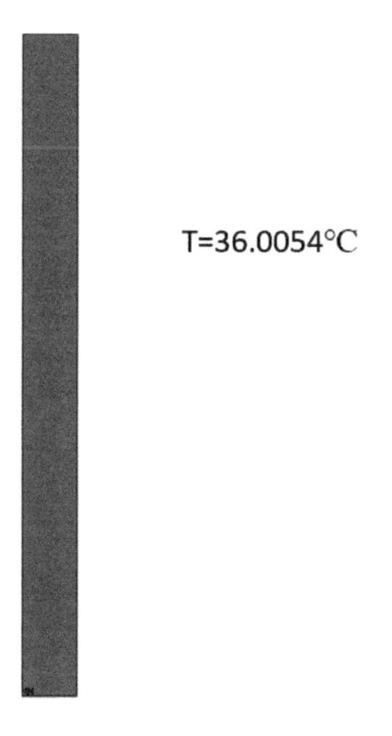

FIGURE 10.5 Temperature distribution (°C).

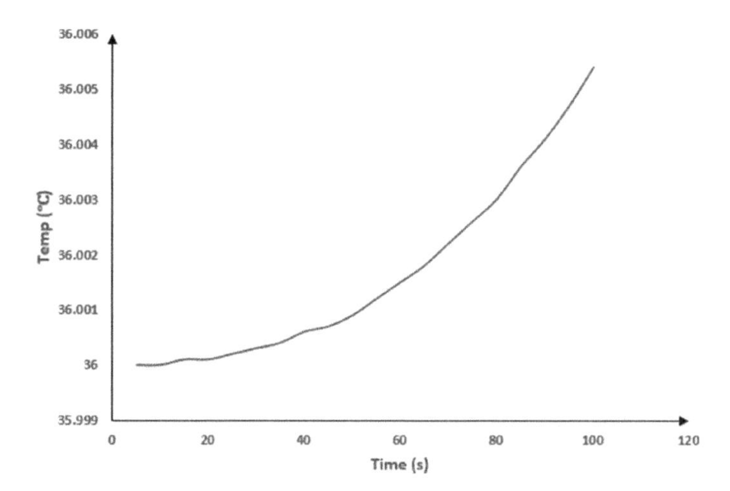

FIGURE 10.6 Temperature change with time.

10.3.6 Discussion

A two-dimensional finite element model was built to simulate heat generation of the biological tissue.

The computational results indicate that with more mechanical energy converted into thermal energy, the temperature increases nonlinearly.

This study includes fully coupled structural-thermal analysis. Therefore, both the structural and thermal boundary conditions and loadings were defined.

In this model, the metric system (kg, mm, s, °C, mA, N, and mV) was selected. Therefore, in the mechanical part, the units for pressure and density became MPa and kg/mm^3, respectively, and in the thermal part, the units for the thermal conductivity and specific heat were mW/(mm K) and mJ/(kg K), respectively.

The material properties are a function of the temperature. Normally, the material parameters should be defined with multiple temperatures in the thermal analysis. In this study, the temperature slightly increases. Thus, one group of the material properties of the biological tissue was specified here.

10.3.7 Summary

Heat generation of the biological tissue was simulated with a fully structural-thermal couple in ANSYS. The temperature increases nonlinearly with more mechanical energy converted into thermal energy.

REFERENCES

1. ANSYS help documentation in the help page of ANSYS190 product.
2. Dill, E.H., *The Finite Element Method for Mechanics of Solids with ANSYS Applications*, CRC Press, Boca Raton, FL, August 2011.
3. Gustafsson, A., *A fibre-reinforced poroviscoelastic finite element model for the Achilles tendon*, Master's Thesis, LUNDS UNIVERSITET, Department of Biomedical Engineering, 2014.
4. Bergstrom, J.S., and Boyce, M.C., "Constitutive modeling of the time-dependent and cyclic loading of elastomers and application to soft biological tissues," *Mechanics of materials*, Vol. 33, 2001, pp. 523–530.

Section III

Coupling among More Than Two Physics Phases

Coupling with more than two physics phases is the topic of Section III. Obviously, it is more difficult to get convergence than coupling between only two physics phases. Therefore, as an example, Section III presents two cases that are solved by the monolithic and partitioned approaches, respectively.

Chapter 11 introduces the CPT elements with an additional temperature degree of freedom and uses it to study arterial tissue fusion.

Blood flow in the abnormal cardiovascular system with two couplings is solved in Chapter 12 with the partitioned approach.

11 Thermal Analysis of Porous Media

Chapter 11 introduces the governing equations for heat transfer in porous media and the finite element modeling procedure in ANSYS. This is followed by a study of arterial tissue fusion.

11.1 GOVERNING EQUATIONS FOR HEAT TRANSFER IN POROUS MEDIA

Biot consolidation with heat transfer contains the solid phase, fluid phase, and thermal phase, which are governed by the different equations. The solid phase follows the force balance equation [1]:

$$\bar{\bar{\nabla}}\boldsymbol{\sigma} - \rho_b \ddot{\mathbf{u}} + \gamma_b \mathbf{g}_v = 0 \tag{11.1}$$

where:

$$\bar{\bar{\nabla}} = \begin{bmatrix} \frac{\partial}{\partial x} & 0 & 0 & \frac{\partial}{\partial y} & 0 & \frac{\partial}{\partial z} \\ 0 & \frac{\partial}{\partial y} & 0 & \frac{\partial}{\partial x} & \frac{\partial}{\partial z} & 0 \\ 0 & 0 & \frac{\partial}{\partial z} & 0 & \frac{\partial}{\partial y} & \frac{\partial}{\partial x} \end{bmatrix} \tag{11.2}$$

ρ_b = bulk density of porous media
$\boldsymbol{\sigma}$ = total Cauchy stress

$$\sigma = \mathbf{D}\varepsilon_{el} - \alpha s_f p\mathbf{I} \tag{11.3}$$

$\mathbf{D}$ = fourth-order elastic tensor
p = pore pressure
α = Biot coefficient
s_f = degree of saturation of fluid
$\mathbf{I}$ = second-order identity tensor
$\mathbf{u}$ = displacement
γ_b = bulk specific weight of porous media
$\mathbf{g}_v$ = gravity load direction

The mass conservation requires that the pore pressure and flow flux of the fluid satisfy the following equation:

$$\nabla \cdot \mathbf{q}_f + \alpha \dot{\varepsilon}_v + \frac{\dot{p}}{Q^*} - s_f \dot{\varepsilon}^{free} = 0 \tag{11.4}$$

where:

$$\nabla = \begin{bmatrix} \frac{\partial}{\partial x} & \frac{\partial}{\partial y} & \frac{\partial}{\partial z} \end{bmatrix}^{\mathrm{T}} \tag{11.5}$$

$\mathbf{q}_f$ = flow flux vector, and

$$= \frac{k_r \mathbf{K}}{\gamma_f}\left(-\nabla p + s_f \gamma_f \mathbf{g}_v\right) \tag{11.6}$$

$\mathbf{K}$ = second-order permeability tensor
k_r = relative permeability
γ_f = specific weight of fluid
ε_v = volumetric strain of the solid skeleton
Q^* = compressibility parameter
ε^{free} = free strain

Thermal transfer in porous media is controlled by:

$$\left(\rho c\right)_{eff} \dot{T} - \nabla \cdot \left(\mathbf{D}_T \nabla T\right) + \nabla \cdot \left(n s_f \rho_f c_f \mathbf{q}_f T\right) = 0 \tag{11.7}$$

where:
$\left(\rho c\right)_{eff}$ = density-specific heat term
$\mathbf{D}_T$ = thermal conductivity
n = porosity
c_f = specific heats of fluid
ρ_f = density of fluid
T = temperature

The porous media is discretized with the following shape functions of the displacement, pressure, and temperature:

$$\mathbf{u} = \mathbf{N}_s^{\mathrm{T}} \mathbf{u}_e \tag{11.8}$$

$$p = \mathbf{N}_p^{\mathrm{T}} \mathbf{p}_e \tag{11.9}$$

$$T = \mathbf{N}_T^{\mathrm{T}} \mathbf{T}_e \tag{11.10}$$

Similar to Equation (4.7), taking the weak form of Equations (11.1, 11.4, and 11.7), and choosing the shape functions as the testing function, yield the matrix form of Equations (11.1, 11.4, and 11.7) [1]:

$$\begin{bmatrix} \mathbf{M}^{ss} & 0 & 0 \\ 0 & 0 & 0 \\ 0 & 0 & 0 \end{bmatrix} \begin{Bmatrix} \ddot{\mathbf{u}} \\ \ddot{\mathbf{p}} \\ \ddot{\mathbf{T}} \end{Bmatrix} + \begin{bmatrix} 0 & 0 & 0 \\ \mathbf{C}^{ps} & \mathbf{C}^{pp} & \mathbf{C}^{pT} \\ 0 & 0 & \mathbf{C}^{TT} \end{bmatrix} \begin{Bmatrix} \dot{\mathbf{u}} \\ \dot{\mathbf{p}} \\ \dot{\mathbf{T}} \end{Bmatrix} + \begin{bmatrix} \mathbf{K}^{ss} & \mathbf{K}^{sp} & \mathbf{K}^{sT} \\ 0 & \mathbf{K}^{pp} & 0 \\ 0 & 0 & \mathbf{K}^{TT} \end{bmatrix} \begin{Bmatrix} \mathbf{u} \\ \mathbf{p} \\ \mathbf{T} \end{Bmatrix} = \begin{Bmatrix} \mathbf{f}^{s} \\ \mathbf{f}^{p} \\ \mathbf{f}^{T} \end{Bmatrix} \tag{11.11}$$

where:

$$\mathbf{M}^{ss} = \int_{\Omega} (\mathbf{N}_s)^{\mathrm{T}} \rho_b \mathbf{N}_s \mathrm{d}\Omega \tag{11.12}$$

$$\mathbf{K}^{ss} = \int_{\Omega} \mathbf{B} \cdot \mathbf{D} \mathbf{B} \mathrm{d}\Omega \tag{11.13}$$

$$\mathbf{K}^{sp} = -\int_{\Omega} \mathbf{B} \cdot \alpha s_f \mathbf{I} \mathbf{N}_p \mathrm{d}\Omega \tag{11.14}$$

$$\mathbf{K}^{sT} = -\int_{\Omega} \mathbf{B} \cdot \mathbf{D} \alpha \mathbf{N}_T \mathrm{d}\Omega \tag{11.15}$$

$$\mathbf{f}^{s} = \int_{\Omega} \mathbf{N}_s \cdot \rho \mathbf{b} \mathrm{d}\Omega + \int_{\Gamma} \mathbf{N}_s \cdot \mathbf{t} \mathrm{d}\Gamma \tag{11.16}$$

$$\mathbf{C}^{ps} = \int_{\Omega} \mathbf{N}_p \cdot \alpha \mathbf{I} \cdot \mathbf{B} \mathrm{d}\Omega \tag{11.17}$$

$$\mathbf{C}^{pp} = \int_{\Omega} \mathbf{N}_p \cdot \frac{1}{Q^*} \mathbf{N}_p \mathrm{d}\Omega \tag{11.18}$$

$$\mathbf{C}^{pT} = -\int_{\Omega} \mathbf{N}_p \cdot s_f \, \beta \mathbf{N}_T \mathrm{d}\Omega \tag{11.19}$$

$$\mathbf{K}^{pp} = \int_{\Omega} \nabla \mathbf{N}_p \cdot \frac{k_r \mathbf{K}}{\gamma_f} \nabla \mathbf{N}_p \mathrm{d}\Omega \tag{11.20}$$

$$\mathbf{f}^{p} = -\int_{\Omega} \mathbf{N}_p \cdot \nabla \cdot \left(\frac{k_r \mathbf{K}}{\gamma_f} s_f \rho_f \mathbf{b} \right) \mathrm{d}\Omega + \int_{\Gamma} \mathbf{N}_p \cdot \mathbf{q} \mathrm{d}\Gamma \tag{11.21}$$

$$\mathbf{C}^{TT} = \int_{\Omega} \mathbf{N}_T \cdot (\rho c)_{eff} \mathbf{N}_T \mathrm{d}\Omega \tag{11.22}$$

$$\mathbf{K}^{TT} = \int_{\Omega} \nabla \mathbf{N}_T \cdot \mathbf{D}_T \nabla \mathbf{N}_T + \mathbf{N}_T \cdot ns_f \rho_f c_f \mathbf{q}_f \nabla \mathbf{N}_T \mathrm{d}\Omega \tag{11.23}$$

$\mathbf{B}$ = strain-displacement operator matrix.

Equations (11.16) and (11.21) are associated with the surface traction $\mathbf{t}$ and flow flux $\mathbf{q}$ at the boundary, respectively.

Equation (11.11) was implemented in ANSYS as a new feature of the CPT elements, which is defined as CPT elements with Keyopt(11)=1 and Keyopt(12)=1 in ANSYS.

11.2 FINITE ELEMENT PROCEDURE FOR CPT THERMAL MODEL

The following points outline the general procedure to build a CPT thermal finite element model:

1. *Build the model*: The model can be built in MADPL and ANSYS Workbench.
2. *Set up the model environment*: CPT elements CPT212/213/215/216/217 with u, p, and T as DOFs are available in ANSYS to build the CPT thermal model. Both Keyopt(11)=1 and Keyopt(12)=1 should be defined to specify p and T as DOFs.
3. *Define the material properties*: In addition to the material properties of porous media, including permeability and the Biot coefficient, the thermal material properties, such as thermal conductivity and specific heat are defined by TB and PM commands in ANSYS.
4. *Mesh the model*: The meshing of porous media is similar to the structural meshing.
5. *Define the boundary conditions and loadings*: The boundary conditions and loadings are specified in ANSYS using SF, D, and BF commands including pore pressure, heat flux, and heat generation.
6. *Solve the equation*: The unsymmetric option for the Newton-Raphson method should be turned on by the commands NROPT, UNSYM because Equation (11.11) is unsymmetrical.
7. *Post-process the analysis*: After solution, the results, including pore pressure, temperature, and heat flux, can be reviewed in both POST1 and POST26 of ANSYS.

11.3 APPLICATION OF CPT THERMAL ELEMENTS FOR STUDY OF ARTERIAL TISSUE FUSION

Some companies have developed devices to fuse blood vessels, but researchers remain unclear about how the tissues respond to the stimuli [2]. Understanding the tissue responses to the heating stimuli is essential for the device design. Therefore, the fusion of biological tissues through heating attracts more and more research interest. Current research has been conducted in both experiments and numerical studies [3]. This study tried to simulate tissue fusion in ANSYS190 using CPT thermal elements.

11.3.1 Finite Element Model

This study simulated an experiment described in [3], in which a flattened artery was clapped within the jaws (Figure 11.1). As it is symmetrical in two directions, one quarter of the finite element model was built to simulate the flattened artery (Figure 11.2a) and meshed with CPT212 (Figure 11.2b) [1]. CPT212 was defined by:

```
ET,1,212
KEYOPT,1,3,2               ! PLANE STRAIN
KEYOPT,1,11,1              ! THERMAL ANALYSIS
KEYOPT,1,12,1              ! PRESSURE DOF
```

To apply the convection condition at the right edge, a thin layer of thermal element 55 was added to connect the CPT elements.

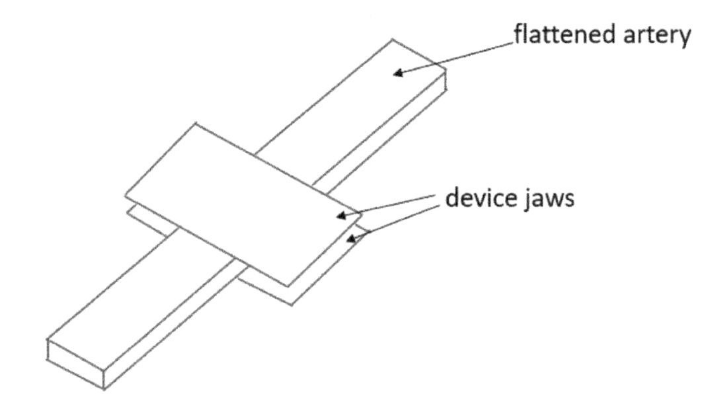

FIGURE 11.1 Schematic of tissue fusion.

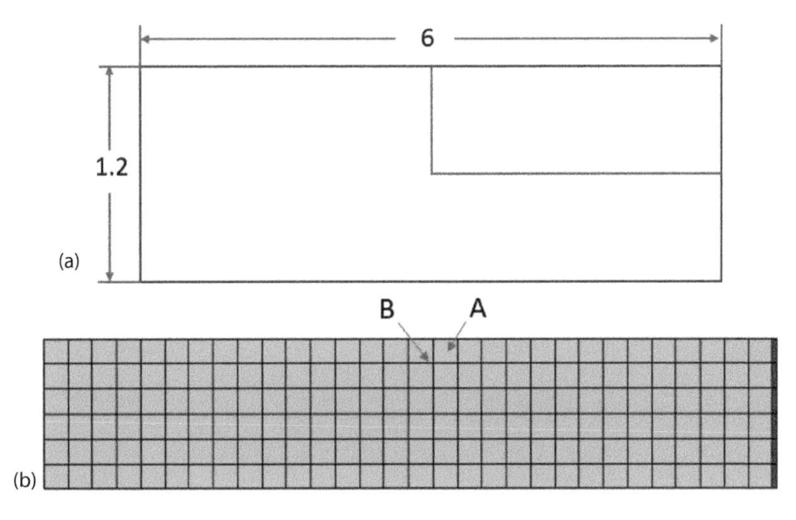

FIGURE 11.2 Finite element model (a) geometry (all dimensions in mm) and (b) finite element model.

TABLE 11.1
Material Properties of the Artery

Young's Modulus (MPa)	Poisson's Ratio	Density (kg/m³)	Permeability (m/s)	Dilatation Coefficient (/°C)	Heat Conductivity (W/m K)	Specific Heat (J/kg K)
6.22	0.3	1050	5e-14	2.5e-4	0.5	146

11.3.2 Material Properties

The material properties of the artery are listed in Table 11.1 and defined in ANSYS by the following commands:

```
MP,EX,1,6.22E6
MP,NUXY,1,0.3
MP,DENS,1,1050

TB,CTE,1
TBDATA,1,2.5E-4,2.5E-4,2.5E-4          ! DILATATION COEFFICIENT

TB,THERM,1,,,COND
TBDATA,1,0.5                           ! HEAT CONDUCTIVITY MATRIX

TB,THERM,1,,,SPHT
TBDATA,1,146                           ! SPECIFIC HEAT

FPX=5E-14
TB,PM,1,,,PERM
TBDATA,1,FPX,FPX,FPX                   ! PERMEABILITY

TB,PM,1,,,BIOT
TBDATA,1,1
```

11.3.3 Boundary and Loadings

The symmetrical conditions were applied on the left edge and the bottom (Figure 11.3). The top edge was loaded with pressure (Figure 11.4) and temperatures from the jaws (Figure 11.5).

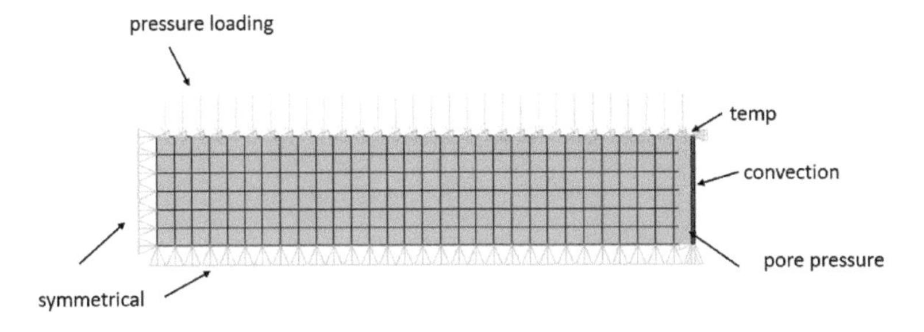

FIGURE 11.3 Boundary conditions and loadings.

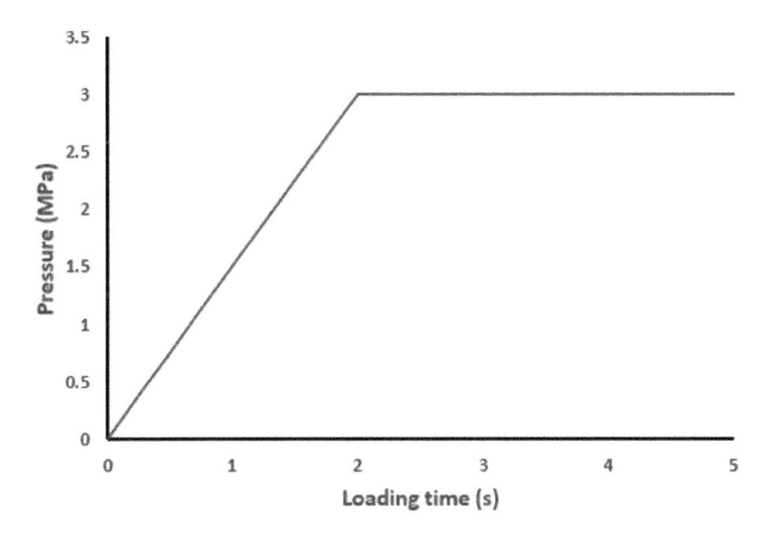

FIGURE 11.4 Pressure loading with time.

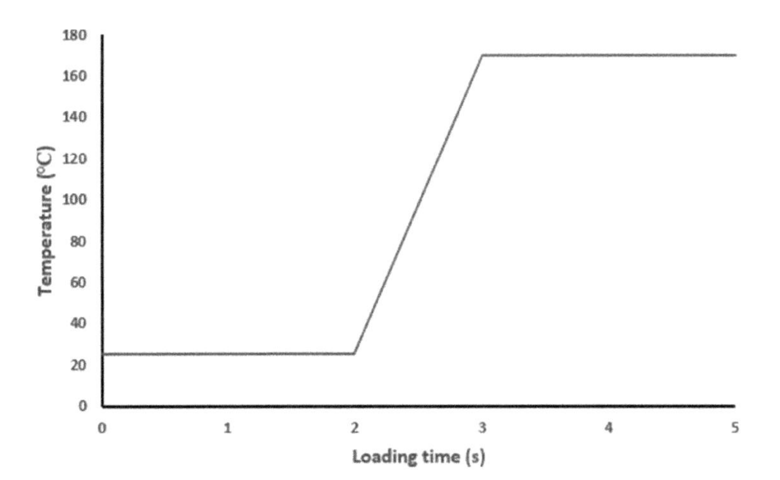

FIGURE 11.5 Temperature loading with time.

```
*DIM,_LOADVARI,TABLE,4,1,1,TIME,
*DIM,_PVARI,TABLE,3,1,1,TIME,

! TIME VALUES
_LOADVARI(1,0,1) = 0.
_LOADVARI(2,0,1) = 2
_LOADVARI(3,0,1) = 3
_LOADVARI(4,0,1) = 5
```

```
! LOAD VALUES
_LOADVARI(1,1,1) = 25
_LOADVARI(2,1,1) = 25
_LOADVARI(3,1,1) = 170
_LOADVARI(4,1,1) = 170

! TIME VALUES
_PVARI(1,0,1) = 0.
_PVARI(2,0,1) = 2
_PVARI(3,0,1) = 5

! LOAD VALUES
_PVARI(1,1,1) = 0
_PVARI(2,1,1) = 3E6
_PVARI(3,1,1) = 3E6

NSEL,S,LOC,Y,H
D,ALL,TEMP,%_LOADVARI%
ALLSEL,ALL
NSEL,S,LOC,Y,H
NSEL,R,LOC,X,0,L
SF,ALL,PRES,%_PVARI%
ALLSEL
```

The right edge allowed water to flow with pore pressure zero.

```
NSEL,S,LOC,X,L
D,ALL,PRES,0
ALLSEL
```

The right edge was also exposed to a convective condition $\left(T_f = 25°\text{C}, h = 25\text{W/m}^2\text{K}\right)$. Thus, the corresponding condition was applied to the thermal elements.

```
NSEL,S,LOC,X,L+LH
SF,ALL,CONV,25,25
ALLSEL
```

11.3.4 Solution Setting

A transient analysis was conducted with NLGEOM, ON to include large deflection effects.

11.3.5 Results

Figure 11.6 shows the final deformation of the tissue. The tissue was compressed in the vertical direction and extended in the horizontal direction. The maximum deformation reached 1.03 mm. The von Mises strains are plotted in Figure 11.7, with the maximum strain 0.42 at the right edge. The von Mises stresses (Figure 11.8) have

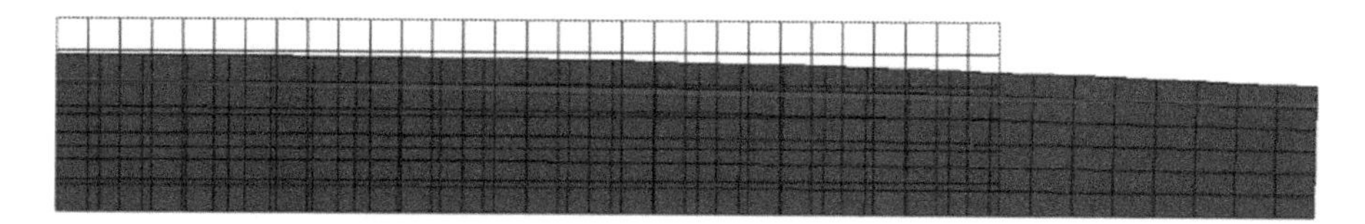

FIGURE 11.6 Deformation of the tissues (m).

FIGURE 11.7 vM strain contour of the tissues.

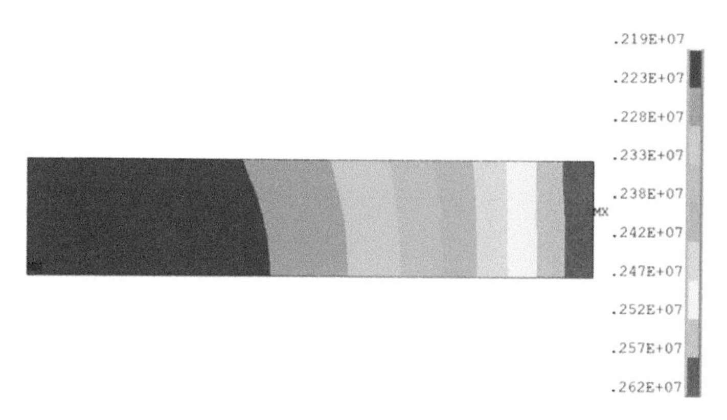

FIGURE 11.8 vM stress contour of the tissues (Pa).

similar distribution, with a peak value 2.62 MPa. Figure 11.9 illustrates the pore pressure distribution. The maximum pore pressure 1.78 MPa occurs at the center. Then, the pore pressure decreases gradually along the horizontal direction until it is zero at the boundary. The final temperature distribution is given in Figure 11.10. The temperature is uniform for the most part except for the area close to the right edge due to the effect of the convection, which matches the reference [3] well. The vertical stress and strain of element A are presented in Figures 11.11 and 11.12, respectively.

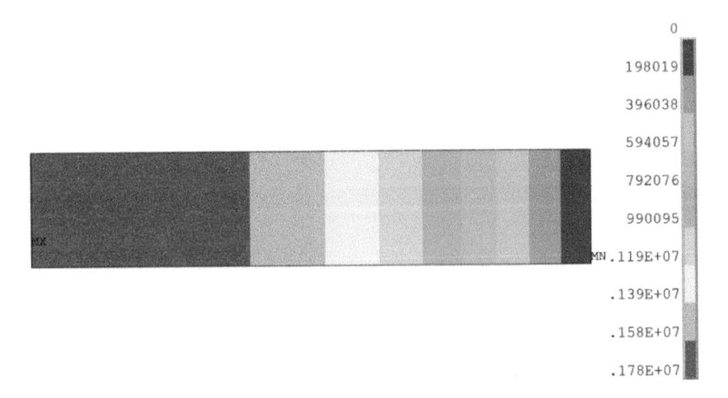

FIGURE 11.9 Pore pressure contour of the tissues (Pa).

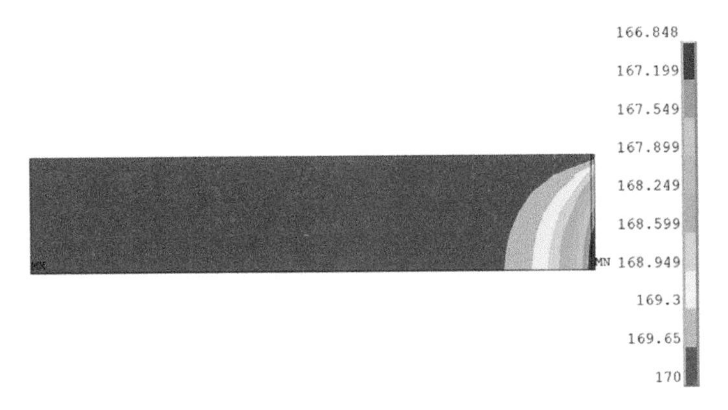

FIGURE 11.10 Temperature distribution of the tissues (°C).

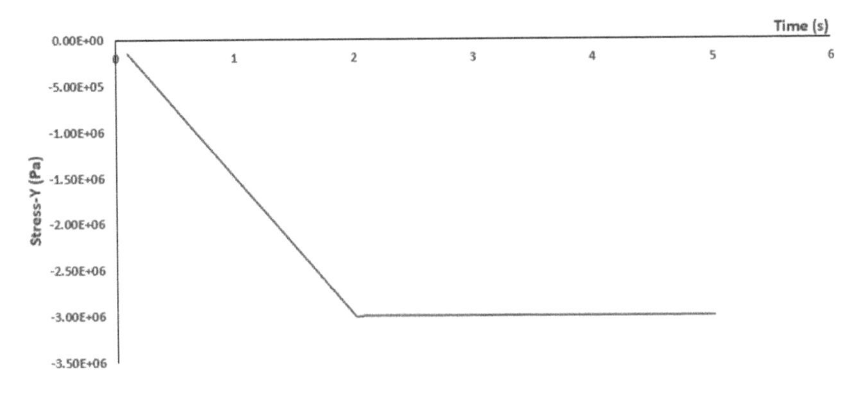

FIGURE 11.11 Vertical stress of element A with time.

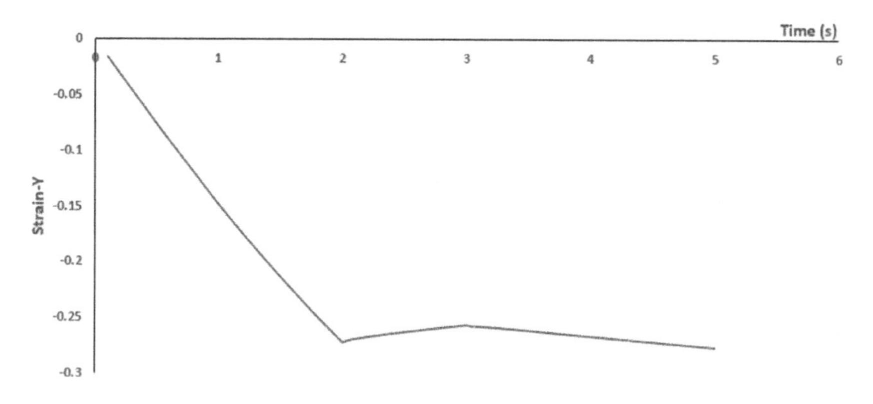

FIGURE 11.12 Vertical strain of element A with time.

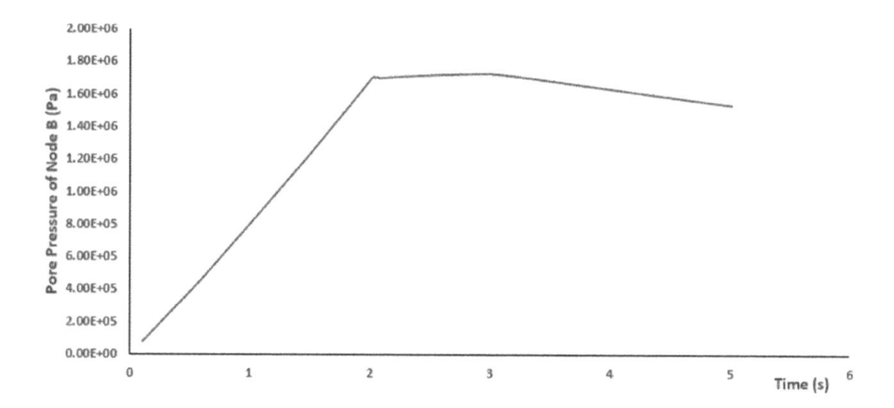

FIGURE 11.13 Pore pressure of node B with time.

The stress results are similar to the loading pressures on the top edge. The vertical strain of element A increases linearly at the beginning, drops a little from time 2 to 3 seconds, and then increases from time 3 to 5 seconds, which matches the reference [3]. Figure 11.13 gives the pore pressure of point B with time.

11.3.6 Discussion

A two-dimensional thermal-porous pressure-coupling finite element model was created to simulate the tissue fusion. The results match the reference, which validate the built model.

Biological tissues, including vertebral disks, arterial tissue, articular cartilage, lung tissue, and tumor, are biphasic and contain the solid and fluid phases. It is appropriate to model them with the CPT elements in ANSYS. When the tissues are under thermal loadings, the thermal option in the CPT elements should be turned on to add a temperature degree of freedom.

The convection cannot be uploaded on the CPT elements directly in ANSYS. Therefore, very thin thermal elements were created at the right edge and connected with the CPT elements. The convection was then loaded on the thermal elements and transferred to the CPT elements. The computational results validate this novel method.

The temperature changes from 25°C to 170°C. Therefore, the material properties of the tissues change with the temperature. Thus, in the model, the material properties, such as Young's modulus should be defined as a function of temperature, which can be implemented by using MPTEMP and MPDATA commands in ANSYS.

11.3.7 Summary

Tissue fusion was modeled in ANSYS using CPT thermal elements. The computational results match the reference, which verifies the built model. Therefore, the built finite element model can be used for further study.

REFERENCES

1. ANSYS help documentation in the help page of ANSYS190 product.
2. Kramer, E.A., and Rentschler, M.E., "Energy-based tissue fusion for sutureless closure: Applications, mechanisms, and potential for function recovery," *Annual Review of Biomedical Engineering*, Vol. 20, 2018, pp. 1–20.
3. Fankell, D.P., Regueiro, R.A., Kramer, E.A., Ferguson, V.L., and Rentschler, M.E., "A small deformation thermoporomechanics finite element model and its application to arterial tissue fusion," *Journal of Mechanical Engineering*, Vol. 140, 2018, p. 031007 (11 pages).

12 A CFD-FEA Coupling Study of Blood Flow in the Abnormal Cardiovascular System

Blood flows in abnormal cardiovascular conditions and generates special sounds called "murmurs" or "bruits" [1]. These sounds can be detected on the skin surface by a stethoscope [2]. It was assumed that disturbances in the blood flow caused by obstruction in the vessels generated the sounds. Thus, the corresponding research has been conducted to study this assumption by means of theoretical analysis [3] and numerical simulation [4]. In this study, this assumption was simulated in ANSYS by computational fluid dynamics-finite element analysis (CFD-FEA) coupling.

12.1 DOUBLE COUPLINGS

A three-dimensional model was built (Figure 12.1) [4], in which two FSI couplings exist (Figure 12.2). The first FSI coupling occurred between the blood flow and the blood vessel. Here, the effect of the vessel deformation on the blood flow was assumed to be negligible. Therefore, the first FSI coupling was simplified as a one-way coupling. The second FSI coupling was defined between the blood vessel and the tissues. Here, the blood vessel was regarded as solid, and the tissues, which are biphasic, were simplified as fluid. Therefore, the second FSI coupling belonged to acoustic FSI. Obviously, the first coupling occurred prior to the second coupling. Thus, the first coupling was analyzed first, and its computational results (pressures on the vessel) were the loadings of the second coupling (Figure 12.3) [4].

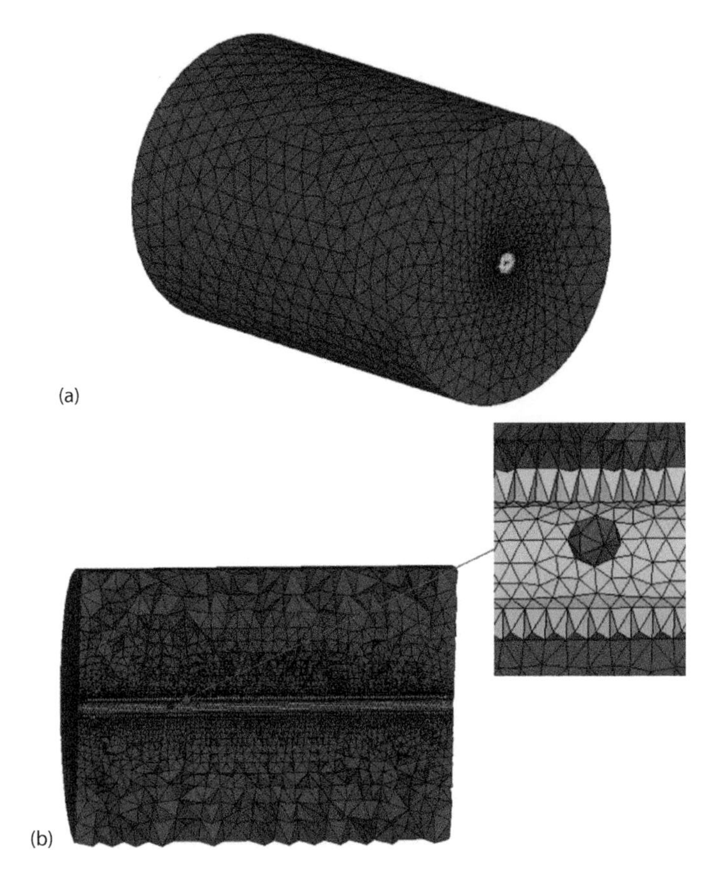

FIGURE 12.1 Finite element model of the abnormal cardiovascular system (a) finite element model and (b) cross section of the model.

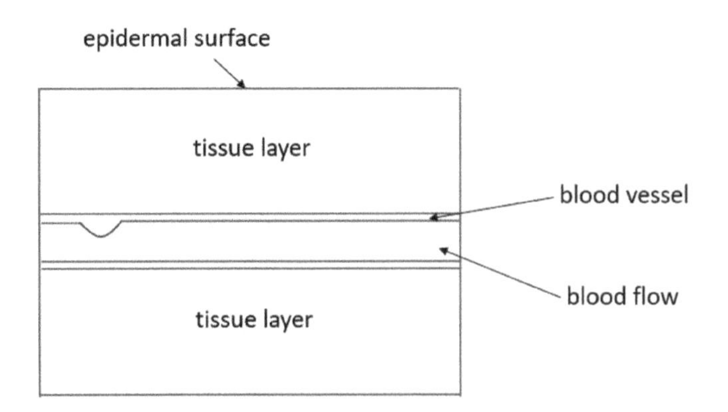

FIGURE 12.2 Schematic of the abnormal cardiovascular system.

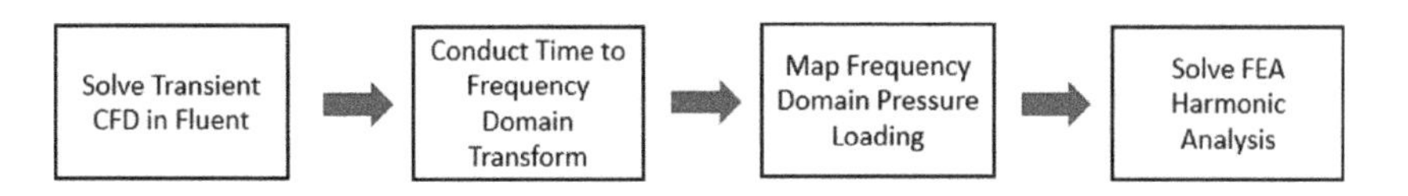

FIGURE 12.3 Solution procedure. (From Khalili, F., *Fluid Dynamics Modeling and Sound Analysis of a Bileaflet Mechanical Heart Valve*, PhD dissertation, University of Central Florida, 2018.)

12.2 BLOOD FLOW IN THE BLOOD VESSEL

The blood flow was driven by a pulsatile pressure drop between the inlet and outlet, which is expressed as [4]:

$$\frac{\Delta P}{\rho v^2} = 0.225 + 1.5 \sin\left(2\pi f t\right) \tag{12.1}$$

where:

$f = 1.25$ Hz
$\rho = 1050$ kg/m^3
$v = 0.59$ m/s

Thus, the pressure defined as a function of time was implemented in the user-defined function (udf) file given in Section 3.4.1.

With the dynamic viscosity as 0.0035 Pa.s, the Reynolds number was set to be 2,000, and the Womersley number as 8.6 [4]. Thus, the flow in the model was defined as laminar.

The CFD analysis was performed in ANSYS Fluent in the following steps:

1. Build geometry of blood vessel and mesh it;
2. Define simulation as transient;
3. Specify the flow as laminar;
4. Define density and dynamic viscosity in the material properties;
5. Specify the pressure at the inlet using the above udf file and outlet as zero;
6. Set up the output of the wall pressure signals on the wall of the blood vessel;
7. Run the transient flow simulation with time step 1 ms to obtain information of high frequencies; and
8. Calculate the Fourier transform of the wall pressure and export the results in the CGNS format.

The details to export the CGNS files are presented in the online video:
www.feabea.net/models/export_CGNS.mp4

12.3 COUPLED ACOUSTIC ANALYSIS OF BLOOD VESSEL AND TISSUES

The coupled acoustic analysis of the blood vessel and tissues was performed in ANSYS MAPDL.

12.3.1 Finite Element Model

The blood vessel was considered as solid and meshed by SOLID185 (Figure 12.1). The tissues were assumed to be fluid and meshed by FLUID30 (Figure 12.1).

12.3.2 Material Properties

The blood vessel was assumed to be linear elastic, with a Young's modulus of 5 MPa and a Poisson's ratio of 0.4. The density and speed of the sound of the vessel were assigned to be 1,200 kg/m^3 and 1,720 m/s, respectively.

12.3.3 Boundary Conditions and Loadings

The fluid pressures by the fluid flow were imported to be applied on the vessel wall using the FLUREAD command:

```
ASEL,S,AREA,,12,13
NSLA,S,1
SF,ALL,FSI          ! DEFINE COUPLE VIBRO-
ACOUSTIC FSI INTERFACE
ALLS
FLUREAD,,FFF_PRESSURE_F5,CGNS,,,,BOTH
! READ ONE-WAY COUPLING CGNS FORMAT FILE
ALLSEL
```

The blood vessel was considered as solid and constrained at the two ends. To allow the vessel to freely expand in the axial directions, MPC contact was applied on the two ends (Figure 12.4). The MPC contact is explained in detail in reference [5].

12.3.4 Solution Setting

Harmonic analysis was conducted in ANSYS190 with a frequency range from 0.2 to 10 Hz.

12.3.5 Results

The acoustic pressures of the skin surface with different frequencies are plotted in Figure 12.5, which have a peak value at frequency around 1.2 Hz. That is consistent

FIGURE 12.4 MPC contact at the end of the artery.

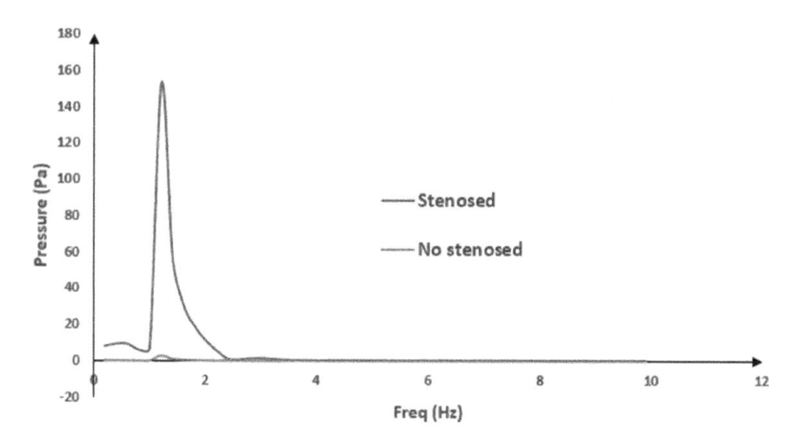

FIGURE 12.5 Acoustic pressures of the skin surface with different frequencies.

with the frequency of the pulsatile pressure in Equation (12.1). Also, it was found that the peak value was much higher than that in cases where the blood vessel had no obstruction, which confirmed the statement that obstruction in the vessels causes the sounds.

Figure 12.6 plots the acoustic pressures of the blood vessel and the tissues at frequency 1.2 Hz, which shows that the acoustic pressures dramatically change in the blood vessel and have nearly uniform distribution in the tissues.

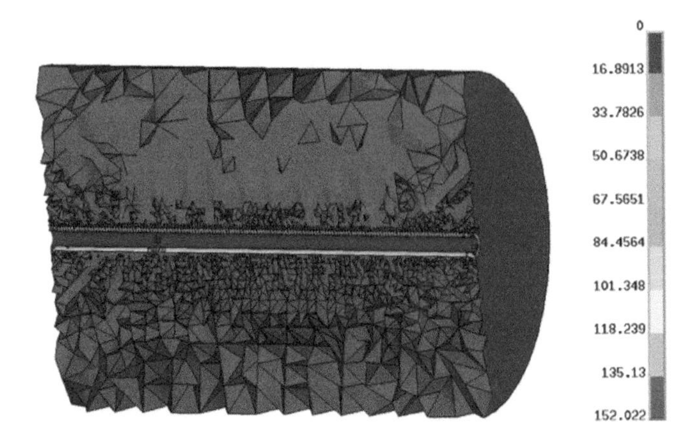

FIGURE 12.6 Acoustic pressure contour (Pa).

12.4 SUMMARY

Blood flows in abnormal cardiovascular conditions were simulated with double couplings. The first coupling occurred between the blood and the vessel wall, and the second coupling existed between the vessel and the tissues. The result of the first coupling was the loading of the second coupling. The computational results indicate that the peak value of the blood vessel with obstruction is much higher than that of the normal blood vessel, which validates that obstruction in the vessels generates the sounds.

REFERENCES

1. Bruns, D.L., "A general theory of the causes of murmurs in the cardiovascular system," *The American Journal of Medicine*, Vol. 27, 1959, pp. 360–374.
2. McKusick, V.A., *Cardiovascular Sound in Health and Disease*, Williams & Wilkins, Baltimore, MD, 1958.
3. Seo, J.H., and Mittal, R., "A coupled flow-acoustic computational study of bruits from a modeled stenosed artery," *Medical & Biological Engineering*, Vol. 50, 2012, pp. 1025–1035.
4. Khalili, F., *Fluid Dynamics Modeling and Sound Analysis of a Bileaflet Mechanical Heart Valve*, PhD dissertation, University of Central Florida, 2018.
5. Yang, Z., *Finite Element Analysis for Biomedical Engineering Applications*, CRC Press, Boca Raton, FL, 2019.

Section IV

Retrospective

The previous three sections discuss modeling of the single physics, coupling between two physics phases, and coupling among more than two physics phases. Section IV summarizes these works and concludes by presenting some rules for modeling coupling problems.

13 Retrospective

Coupling is very complicated because it occurs among different physics phases. The previous three parts lead to the following conclusions:

1. *Influence of natures of various phases of physics on physical modeling*: The natures of various phases of physics significantly influence the physical modeling. A solid keeps a constant shape and has finite deformation under external loadings. Therefore, it adopts the Lagrangian description and studies the stress and strain of one material point. Unlike solids, fluid can flow freely. Thus, fluid uses the Eulerian description and focuses on the velocity and pressure of the whole domain. Sound is a wave governed by the wave equation, while heat flows in the media following the heat transfer equation.

   The physical models have different degrees of freedom. Accordingly, their modeling procedures change in ANSYS, which is summarized in Table 13.1.
2. *Problem-dependent coupling methods*: Coupling refers to a combination of different physical domains. Selecting coupling methods depends upon the specific problems. Because every phase of physics has its unique features, coupling problems are very difficult to solve. Therefore, different coupling methods may be chosen for various coupling problems. In this book, the one-way coupling and two-way coupling were used for fluid-structure interaction (FSI), while the acoustic FSI and thermal-structural coupling adopt the monolithic approach in which the structural equations and thermal equations/acoustic equations are integrated and solved simultaneously.
3. *Special meshing requirement for various physical models*: Various physical models have different meshing requirements. The solid model needs fine meshing at the high stress gradient, while fluid requires fine meshing at the boundary because of the boundary layer. At the highest working frequency in the acoustic field, obtaining a reliable solution demands either ten elements per wavelength for low-order elements or five elements per wavelength for high-order elements. The monolithic approach requires the identical meshing for the coupling domains, but it is not necessary for one-way coupling and two-way coupling.
4. *Units for coupling problems*: Coupling problems involve different physical domains, which are associated with different units. To make the units consistent, it would be a good choice to select the SI units (kg, m, s, K, A, N, and V).

TABLE 13.1
DOFs and Boundary Conditions and Loadings of Various Physical Models

Physical Domains	DOFs	Elements in ANSYS	Boundary Conditions and Loadings
Solid	u	181/182/183/185/186/187/188/189	Displacement, force, et al.
Fluid	V, p		Pressure, velocity, et al.
Thermal	T	70/77/87/292/278 /279/291	Temperature, heat flux, et al.
Acoustic	P	29/30/220/221	Acoustic pressure, et al.
Porous media	u, p	212/213/215/216/217	Porous pressure, displacement, force, et al.
Thermal structural	u, T	222/223/226/227 with Keyopt(1)=11	Displacement, force, temperature, heat flux, et al.
Acoustic FSI	u, p	30/220/221 with Keyopt(2)=0	Displacement, acoustic pressure, et al.
Porous thermal	u, p, T	212/213/215/216/217 with Keyopt(11)=1	Displacement, porous pressure, temperature, heat flux, et al.

Appendix 1

Input File of IVD Model in Section 2.4

```
/PREP7
/COM, UNITS (N, MM, MPA,  S)
/COM,  GEOMETRY
K,    3,  82.6-68,      47.9
K,    2,  78.0-68,      45.1
K,    1,  0,      42.8
K,    4,  83.0-68,      53.7
K,    5,  79.7-68,      57.6
K,    7,  0,      58.5
K,    6,  73.3-68,      60.0
K,    12,  92.4-68,      50.5
K,    9,  80.2-68,      35.1
K,   16,  73.3-68,      67.4
K,   14,  86.3-68,      64.5
K,   10,  84.7-68,      38.2
K,   13,  80.1-68,      67.0
K,   17,  0,         65.6
K,   11,  90.0-68,      45.2
K,   15,  90.6-68,      58.1
K,  8,  0,      31.9
KSEL, S, KP, , 1, 7
BSPLINE, ALL
KSEL, S, KP, , 8, 17
BSPLINE, ALL
ALLSEL
LSTR,    17,     7
LSTR,     7,     1
LSTR,     1,    8

AL, 1, 4
AL, 2, 3, 1, 5

W=1
E1=1.5

ET, 1, 182
ESIZE, W
AMESH, 1, 2
ET, 2, 185
```

```
ESIZE, , 2
VEXT, 1, 2, 1, , , 5
ESIZE, , 5
VEXT, 3, 6, 3, , , 10
ESIZE, , 2
VEXT, 10, 13, 3, , , 5
ALLSEL

ACLEAR, 1, 2
ALLSEL

/COM,  MATERIAL PROPERTIES
! BONE
MP, EX, 1, 3500                !MPA
MP, NUXY, 1, 0.3

!NUCLEUS
MP, EX, 2, E1/10
MP, NUXY, 2, 0.17

!ANNULUS
MP, EX, 3, E1
MP, NUXY, 3, 0.17

VSEL, S, VOLU, , 3
ESLV, S
EMODIF, ALL, MAT, 2
ALLSEL

VSEL, S, VOLU, , 4
ESLV, S
EMODIF, ALL, MAT, 3
ALLSEL

/COM,  BOUNDARY CONDITIONS
NSEL, S, LOC, Z
D, ALL, UZ, 0
ALLSEL
NSEL, S, LOC, X
D, ALL, UX, 0
ALLSEL

NSEL, S, LOC, Z, 20
SF, ALL, PRES, 0.5
ALLSEL

D, NODE(0, 65.6, 0), UY, 0
ALLSEL

FINISH
```

```
/SOLU
NLGEOM, ON
OUTRES, ALL, ALL
TIME, 1
NSUBST, 5
SOLVE

NSEL, S, LOC, Z, 20
SF, ALL, PRES, 0
ALLSEL
SOLV

FINI
```

Appendix 2

Input File of Acoustic Model in Section 4.4

```
/COM, THIS MODEL CAN BE REPEATED INTO ANSYS190 AND
LATER VERSIONS
/PREP7
/COM,  UNITS (N,  M,  PA,  S)
E_SIZE=0.1
RECTNG, -10, 10, -10, 10
RECTNG, -9.5, 9.5, -9.5, 9.5
RECTNG, -9.5, -4, -9.5, -4
AOVLAP, 1, 2, 3
WPOFF, 3, 3
CYL4, 0, 0, 0.5
ASBA,       5,        1
WPOFF, -3, -3
AGLUE, ALL

ET, 1, MESH200, 7
ET, 2, MESH200, 7
ET, 3, FLUID220, , 1                    ! UNCOUPLED
ET, 4, FLUID220, , 1, , 1               ! PML

MP, DENS, 1, 1.030                      ! DENSITY
MP, SONC, 1, 340                        ! SONIC VELOCITY
ESIZE, E_SIZE
TYPE, 2
AMESH, 2, 4, 2
TYPE, 1
AMESH, 6

TYPE, 3
ESIZE, , 1
VEXT, 2, 4, 2, 0, 0, E_SIZE
ALLSEL
TYPE, 4
ESIZE, , 1
VEXT, 6, , , 0, 0, E_SIZE
ALLSEL
```

```
ACLEAR, ALL
ETDELE, 1
ETDELE, 2
ALLSEL
NUMMRG, NODE
ALLSEL

NSEL, S, LOC, X, -4
NSEL, R, LOC, Y, -4
BF, ALL, MASS, 0.01                 ! MASS SOURCE
ALLSEL
FINI

/SOLU
EQSLV, SPARSE
ANTYPE, HARMIC                      ! HARMONIC ANALYSIS
HROPT, FULL
HARFRQ, , 500
NSUB, 50
SOLVE
FINI

/POST1
SET, 1, 50, , AMPL             ! PLOT THE ACOUSTIC PRESSURE
PLNSOL, SPL                    ! ACOUSTIC PRESSURE - DBA

/POST26
NUMVAR, 200
NSOL, 3, 1573, SPL
NSOL, 4, 1546, SPL
PRVAR, 3, 4
```

Appendix 3

Input File of Model of Breast Tumor in Section 5.4

```
/PREP7
/COM, UNITS (N, M, PA, S, K)
PI=3.1416
/COM,  MATERIAL PROPERTIES
MP, C, 1, 3000
MP, KXX, 1, 0.42
MP, DENS, 1, 920

MP, C, 2, 3800
MP, KXX, 2, 0.42
MP, DENS, 2, 1052

/COM,  GEOMETRY
PCIRC,  , 0.09, 0, 180,
CYL4, -0.0115, 0.0623,  ,  , 0.0115, 360
AOVLAP, ALL

ESIZE, 0.02*0.09
ET, 1, 55
MAT, 2
AMESH, 2
MAT, 1
ESIZE, 0.05*0.09
AMESH, 3
ALLSEL

ESEL, S, MAT, , 1
NSLE, S
*GET, NNUM_N1, NODE, 0, COUNT
VOL_1=(PI*0.09**2/2-PI*0.0115**2)/NNUM_N1
ALLSEL
ESEL, S, MAT, , 2
NSLE, S
*GET, NNUM_N2, NODE, 0, COUNT
VOL_2=PI*0.0115**2/NNUM_N2
ALLSEL

/COM,  ELEMENT DEFINITION
ET, 2, 71, , , 1, 1
R, 2, VOL_1*496.8, (35.8+273), -1
```

```
ET, 3, 71, , , 1, 1
R, 3, VOL_2*35978, (36.8+273), -1

/COM,  CONVECTION
SFL, 1, CONV, 10,  , 20+273,

LSEL, S, LINE, , 1
NSLL, S, 1
CM, N1, NODE
ALLSEL
TOFFST, 0
ALLSEL
D, NODE(0, 0, 0), TEMP, 35.8+273
ALLSEL

ESEL, S, MAT, , 2
NSLE, S
CM, N2, NODE
ALLSEL

/COM,  INITIAL TEMPERATURES OF NODES
CMSEL, U, N1, NODE
CMSEL, U, N2, NODE
*GET, NNUM_N, NODE, 0, COUNT ! GET NUMBER OF NODES
*GET, N_MIN, NODE, 0, NUM, MIN ! GET MIN NODE NUMBER

*DO, I, 1, NNUM_N, 1 ! OUTPUT TO ASCII BY LOOPING OVER NODES
CURR_N=N_MIN
TYPE, 2
REAL, 2
E, CURR_N
IC, CURR_N, TEMP, 35.8+273
*GET, N_MIN, NODE, CURR_N, NXTH
*ENDDO
ALLSEL

CMSEL, S, N2, NODE
*GET, NNUM_N, NODE, 0, COUNT ! GET NUMBER OF NODES
*GET, N_MIN, NODE, 0, NUM, MIN ! GET MIN NODE NUMBER
*DO, J, 1, NNUM_N, 1 ! OUTPUT TO ASCII BY LOOPING OVER NODES
CURR_N=N_MIN
TYPE, 3
REAL, 3
E, CURR_N
IC, CURR_N, TEMP, 36.8+273
*GET, N_MIN, NODE, CURR_N, NXTH
*ENDDO
ALLSEL

CMSEL, S, N1, NODE
IC, ALL, TEMP, 273+35.8
```

```
ALLSEL
FINISH
/SOL
TIME, 1000
ANTYPE, 4
NSUBST, 1000, 3000, 1000
OUTRES, ALL, ALL
SOLV
FINI

/POST1
/EFACET, 1
SET, 1, LAST
PLNSOL,  TEMP, ,  0
FLST, 2, 2, 1
FITEM, 2, 259
FITEM, 2, 290
PATH, 12, 2, 30, 20,
PPATH, P51X, 1
PDEF, 22, TEMP,  , AVG
/PBC, PATH,  , 0
PLPATH, 22                 ! TEMPERATURE ON PATH AB
PRPATH, 22
```

Appendix 4

UDF File in Section 7.2

```
/************************************************************
vprofile.c
UDF for specifying unsteady-state velocity profile boundary
condition
************************************************************/
#include "udf.h"
DEFINE_PROFILE(inlet_x_velocity, thread, position)
{
  real x[ND_ND]; /* this will hold the position vector */
  real r, d;
  face_t f;
  real velocity_mag;
  real t=CURRENT_TIME;
  r = 0.01; /* inlet height in m */
if ((t>=0.0) && (t<0.25))
{
velocity_mag=0.015+t*0.1;
}
if ((t>=0.25) && (t<0.4))
{
velocity_mag=0.04+0.440/0.15*(t-0.25);
}
if ((t>=0.4) && (t<1.0))
{
velocity_mag=0.480-0.460/0.6*(t-0.4);
}
if ((t>=1.0) && (t<1.25))
{
velocity_mag=0.015+(t-1)*0.1;
}
if ((t>=1.25) && (t<1.4))
{
velocity_mag=0.04+0.440/0.15*(t-1.25);
}
if ((t>=1.4) && (t<2.0))
{
velocity_mag=0.480-0.460/0.6*(t-1.4);
}
if ((t>=2.0) && (t<2.25))
```

```
{
velocity_mag=0.015+(t-2)*0.1;
}
if ((t>=2.25) && (t<2.4))
{
velocity_mag=0.04+0.440/0.15*(t-2.25);
}
if ((t>=2.4) && (t<3.0))
{
velocity_mag=0.480-0.460/0.6*(t-2.4);
}
  begin_f_loop(f,thread)
  {
    F_CENTROID(x, f, thread);
     /* non-dimensional d coordinate */
    d = ((x[0]+0.0079)*(x[0]+0.0079)+x[2]*x[2])/r/r;
    F_PROFILE(f, thread, position) = velocity_mag*(1.0-d);
  }
  end_f_loop(f, thread)
}
```

Appendix 5

Input File of Model of Confined Compression Test in Section 8.3

```
/PREP7
/COM,  UNITS (N,  MM,  MPA,  S)
ET, 1, CPT212
KEYOPT, 1, 3, 1                               ! AXISYMMETRICAL
KEYOPT, 1, 12, 1                              ! DOF P
C1=0.015                                      ! MPA

MP, EX, 1, C1
MP, NUXY, 1, 0.49

FPX=8E-2                                      ! MM^4/N.S
ONE=1.0
TB, PM, 1, , , PERM
TBDATA, 1, FPX
TB, PM, 1, , , BIOT                           ! BIOT COEFFICIENT
TBDATA, 1, ONE

A=2                                           ! MM
B=10                                          ! MM

RECTNG,  0,  A,  0,  B

ESIZE, 0.2
AMESH, 1

ALLSEL
NSEL, S, LOC, X, 0
NSEL, A, LOC, X, A
D, ALL, UX
ALLSEL

NSEL, S, LOC, Y, 0
D, ALL, UY, 0
D, ALL, PRES, 0
ALLSEL
```

```
NSEL, S, LOC, Y, B
SF, ALL, PRES, 0.001                          !MPA
ALLSEL

FINISH

/SOLU
NLGEOM, ON
KBC, 1                                        !STEPPED LOADING
TIME, 1E4
NSUBST, 200, 1000, 50

OUTRES, ALL, ALL
SOLVE

FINISH

/POST26
NSOL, 2, 70, U, Y
PLVAR, 2
```

Appendix 6

Input File of Ear Model in Section 9.3

```
/COM, THIS MODEL CAN BE REPEATED INTO ANSYS190 AND
LATER VERSIONS
/PREP7
/COM,  UNITS (N,  M,  PA,  S)
/COM,  GEOMETRY
CONE, 6E-3, 4.5E-3, 0, 21E-3, 0, 360,
CONE, 4.5E-3, 4.5E-3, 21E-3, 25E-3, 0, 360,
CONE, 4.5E-3, 5.5E-3, 25E-3, 36E-3, 0, 360,
WPOFFS, , , 25E-3
WPROTA, , -30
BLOCK, -10E-3, 10E-3, -10E-3, 10E-3, 0, 0.25E-3,
VGLUE, 1, 2, 3
VOVLAP, 4, 5, 6
VDELE, 11
ALLSEL
VPLOT

/COM,  MATERIAL PROPERTIES
ALPHA=0.66
TAU=25E-6
MP, EX, 1, 23E6
MP, NUXY, 1, 0.3
MP, DENS, 1, 1200
TB, PRONY, 1, , 1, SHEAR
TBDATA, 1, ALPHA, TAU

TB, PRONY, 1, , 1, BULK
TBDATA, 1, ALPHA, TAU

MP, DENS, 2, 1.21
MP, SONC, 2, 343

/COM,  ELEMENT TYPES
ET, 1, SOLID187
ET, 2, FLUID221, , 1

MSHAPE, 1, 3D
ESIZE, 1E-3
TYPE, 1
MAT, 1
```

```
VMESH, 7, 10, 3
ALLSEL

TYPE, 2
MAT, 2
VSEL, U, VOLU, , 7, 10, 3
VMESH, ALL

/COM,  BOUNDARY CONDITIONS AND LOADINGS
ASEL, S, AREA, , 30, 32
ASEL, A, AREA, , 24
NSLA, S, 1
D, ALL, UX, , , , , UY, UZ
ALLSEL

*DIM, _LOADVARI, TABLE, 3, 1, 1, TIME,
! TIME VALUES
_LOADVARI(1, 0, 1) = 0.
_LOADVARI(2, 0, 1) = 0.5E-3
_LOADVARI(3, 0, 1) = 2E-3

! LOAD VALUES
_LOADVARI(1, 1, 1) = 1E4.
_LOADVARI(2, 1, 1) = 0
_LOADVARI(3, 1, 1) = 0

ASEL, S, AREA, , 1
NSLA, S, 1
D, ALL, PRES, %_LOADVARI%
ALLSEL

ECPCHG
FINISH

/SOLU
ANTYPE, 4      ! TRANSIENT ANALYSIS
EQSLV, SPARSE
KBC, 1
OUTRES, ALL, ALL
NSUBST, 250, 3000, 50
TIME, 2E-3
SOLV
FINISH

/POST26
NSOL, 2, 1683, PRES
NSOL, 3, 746, PRES
NSOL, 4, 32918, PRES
PLVAR, 2, 3, 4
NSOL, 5, 908, U, Z,
PLVAR, 5
```

Appendix 7

Input File of Model of Soft Tissues in Section 10.3

```
/COM, THIS MODEL CAN BE REPEATED INTO ANSYS194 AND LATER
VERSIONS
/BATCH, LIST
/COM,  UNITS(N,  MM,  MPA,  S,  K)

LX=0.73          ! LENGTH,  MM
LY=8.51          ! WIDTH,  MM

! MATERIAL PARAMETERS FOR BERGSTROM-BOYCE MODEL
MUA=100          ! INITIAL SHEAR MODULUS FOR PART A  (MPA)
NA=2.62*2.62     ! SQUARE OF LIMITING CHAIN STRAIN FOR PART A
MUB=100          ! INITIAL SHEAR MODULUS FOR PART B (MPA)
NB=2.62*2.62     ! SQUARE OF LIMITING CHAIN STRAIN FOR PART B
C5=0.18          ! CREEP MATERIAL CONSTANT
C6=-0.16         ! CREEP MATERIAL CONSTANT
C7=1.79          ! CREEP MATERIAL CONSTANT
INVK=1/5000      ! INVERSE OF THE BULK MODULUS

RHO=1.67E-6      ! DENSITY  KG/MM^3
KT=0.42          ! THERMAL CONDUCTIVITY  MW/(MM.K)
CT=3000E3        ! SPECIFIC HEAT CAPACITY MJ/(KG.K)
QR=0.9           ! QRATE

/PREP7
ET, 1, 223, 11     ! STRUCTURAL-THERMAL ANALYSIS
KEYOPT, 1, 9, 1
KEYOPT, 1, 3, 1

RECT, 0, LX, 0, LY
ESIZE, LX/2
TYPE, 1
AMESH, 1

TB, BB, 1, , , ISO
TBDATA, 1, MUA
TBDATA, 2, NA
TBDATA, 3, MUB
TBDATA, 4, NB
TBDATA, 5, C5
TBDATA, 6, C6
TBDATA, 7, C7
```

```
MP, DENS, 1, RHO
MP, KXX, 1, KT
MP, C, 1, CT

MP, QRATE, 1, QR

NSEL, S, LOC, X, 0
D, ALL, UX, 0
NSEL, ALL

NSEL, S, LOC, Y, 0
D, ALL, UY, 0
NSEL, ALL

IC, ALL, TEMP, 36
TREF, 0
FINI
/SOLU
ANTYPE, 4
NLGEOM, ON
KBC, 0
OUTRES, ALL, LAST
*DO, I, 1, 10
TIME, (I-1)*10+5
NSEL, S, LOC, Y, LY
SF, ALL, PRES, -I       ! MPA
ALLSEL
NSUBST, 100, 1000, 30
/OUT, SCRATCH
SOLVE
TIME, (I-1)*10+10
NSEL, S, LOC, Y, LY
SF, ALL, PRES, 0
ALLSEL
NSUBST, 100, 1000, 30
SOLVE
*ENDDO

/OUT
FINI

/POST26
NSOL, 2, 46, TEMP
PRVAR, 2
```

Appendix 8

Input File of Tissue Fusion in Section 11.3

```
/COM, THIS MODEL CAN BE REPEATED INTO ANSYS190 AND LATER
VERSIONS
/PREP7
/COM,  UNITS (N,  M,  PA,  S,  K)
H=0.6E-3
L=3E-3
LH=0.02E-3
ET, 1, 212
KEYOPT, 1, 3, 2
KEYOPT, 1, 11, 1                     ! THERMAL STUDY ON
KEYOPT, 1, 12, 1                     ! PRESSURE DOF ON

MP, EX, 1, 6.22E6
MP, NUXY, 1, 0.3
MP, DENS, 1, 1050

TB, CTE, 1
TBDATA, 1, 2.5E-4, 2.5E-4, 2.5E-4    ! DILATATION COEFFICIENT

TB, THERM, 1, , , COND
TBDATA, 1, 0.5                       ! HEAT CONDUCTIVITY MATRIX

TB, THERM, 1, , , SPHT
TBDATA, 1, 146                       ! SPECIFIC HEAT

FPX=5E-14
TB, PM, 1, , , PERM
TBDATA, 1, FPX, FPX, FPX             ! SOLID PERMEABILITY

TB, PM, 1, , , BIOT
TBDATA, 1, 1

RECTNG, 0, L, 0, H
RECTNG, L, L+LH, 0, H
AGLUE, ALL

TYPE, 1
MAT, 1
```

```
ESIZE, 0.1E-3
AMESH, 1

ET, 2, 55
MP, C, 2, 146
MP, KXX, 2, 0.5
MP, DENS, 2, 1000

TYPE, 2
MAT, 2
AMESH, 3

NSEL, S, LOC, X, 0
D, ALL, UX, 0
SF, ALL, HFLUX, 0
NSEL, S, LOC, Y, 0
D, ALL, UY, 0
SF, ALL, HFLUX, 0
ALLSEL

NSEL, S, LOC, X, L
D, ALL, PRES, 0                          !PORE PRESSURE 0
ALLSEL

NSEL, S, LOC, X, L+LH
SF, ALL, CONV, 25, 25                     !CONVECTION
ALLSEL

*DIM, _LOADVARI, TABLE, 4, 1, 1, TIME,
*DIM, _PVARI, TABLE, 3, 1, 1, TIME,

! TIME VALUES
_LOADVARI(1, 0, 1) = 0.
_LOADVARI(2, 0, 1) = 2
_LOADVARI(3, 0, 1) = 3
_LOADVARI(4, 0, 1) = 5

! LOAD VALUES
_LOADVARI(1, 1, 1) = 25
_LOADVARI(2, 1, 1) = 25
_LOADVARI(3, 1, 1) = 170
_LOADVARI(4, 1, 1) = 170

! TIME VALUES
_PVARI(1, 0, 1) = 0.
_PVARI(2, 0, 1) = 2
_PVARI(3, 0, 1) = 5
```

```
! LOAD VALUES
_PVARI(1, 1, 1) = 0
_PVARI(2, 1, 1) = 3E6
_PVARI(3, 1, 1) = 3E6

IC, ALL, TEMP, 25
TREF, 25
FINISH

/SOLU

ANTYPE, TRANS
TIME, 5
NLGEOM, ON
NSEL, S, LOC, Y, H
D, ALL, TEMP, %_LOADVARI%
ALLSEL, ALL
NSEL, S, LOC, Y, H
NSEL, R, LOC, X, 0, L
SF, ALL, PRES, %_PVARI%
ALLSEL

OUTRES, ALL, ALL
NSUBST, 50, 1000, 30
KBC, 0
SOLV

FINISH
```

Appendix 9

Input File of Blood Flow Model in Section 12.3

```
/COM, DOWNLOAD  FFF_PRESSURE_F5.cgns FROM
/COM, www.feabea.net/models/ FFF_PRESSURE_F5.cgns
/COM, DOWNLOAD  FFF_PRESSURE_F5_1.cgns FROM
/COM, www.feabea.net/models/ FFF_PRESSURE_F5_1.cgns
/COM, THIS MODEL CAN BE REPEATED INTO ANSYS190 AND LATER
VERSIONS
/PREP7
/COM,  UNITS (N,  M,  PA,  S)
/COM,  GEOMETRY
D=12E-3
L=30*D
CYLIND, D/2,  , 0, L, 0, 360,
WPOFF, 0, 0, 0.09
SPH4, 0, 0.006, 0.003
VSBV,       1,       2
WPOFF, 0, 0, -0.09
CYLIND, D*0.8, 0, 0, L, 0, 360,
VSBV,       1,       3

CYLIND, D*10.8,  D*0.8, 0, L, 0, 360,
VGLUE, ALL

ET, 1, 185
ET, 2, 30
ET, 3, 154            ! SURFACE ELEMENT
ET, 4, 30, , , , , 1

/COM,  MATERIAL PROPERTIES
MP, DENS, 1, 1100
MP, EX, 1, 5E6
MP, NUXY, 1, 0.4
MP, DENS, 2, 1200
MP, SONC, 2, 1720
MP, VISC, 2, 1E-4
MP, EX, 3, 2.19E6
MP, NUXY, 3, 0.39
MP, DENS, 3, 1450
```

```
TYPE, 1
MAT, 1
ESIZE, 0.2*D
MSHAPE, 1, 3D
VMESH, 3

TYPE, 2
MAT, 2
ESIZE, 2*D
VMESH, 1
ALLSEL

NSEL, S, NODE, , NODE(-0.15634E-003, 0.30848E-002, 0.90691E-
001)
ESLN, S
NSLE, S
ESLN, S
ESEL, R, CENT, X, -0.29E-2, 0.29E-2
ESEL, R, CENT, Z, 0.087, 0.093
ESEL, R, CENT, Y, 0.31E-2, 0.60E-2
EMODIF, ALL, MAT, 3
ALLSEL

/COM,  MPC CONTACT AT TWO ENDS OF VESSEL
MAT, 1
R, 13
REAL, 13
ET, 13, 170
ET, 14, 174
KEYOPT, 14, 12, 5
KEYOPT, 14, 4, 1
KEYOPT, 14, 2, 2
KEYOPT, 13, 2, 1
KEYOPT, 13, 4, 111111
TYPE, 13
N, 1E6, 0, 0, 0.36
N, 1E6+1, 0, 0, 0
TSHAP, PILOT
TYPE, 13
REAL, 13
E, 1E6

TYPE, 14
REAL, 13
ASEL, S, AREA, , 15
NSLA, S, 1
ESLN, S
ESURF
```

```
MAT, 1
R, 14
REAL, 14
ET, 15, 170
ET, 16, 174
KEYOPT, 16, 12, 5
KEYOPT, 16, 4, 1
KEYOPT, 16, 2, 2
KEYOPT, 15, 2, 1
KEYOPT, 15, 4, 111111

TSHAP, PILOT
TYPE, 15
REAL, 14
E, 1E6+1

TYPE, 16
REAL, 14
ASEL, S, AREA, , 14
NSLA, S, 1
ESLN, S
ESURF

NSEL, S, NODE, , 1E6, 1E6+1
D, ALL, ALL
ALLSEL

ESEL, S, CENT, Z, 0.32, 0.36
ESEL, A, CENT, Z, 0, 0.04
ESEL, R, TYPE, , 2
EMODIF, ALL, TYPE, 4
ALLSEL

ASEL, S, AREA, , 7, 8
ASEL, A, AREA, , 4
NSLA, S, 1
TYPE, 3
ESURF
ALLSEL
ESEL, S, TYPE, , 3
NSLE, S
SF, ALL, FSIN, 1
ALLSEL

ASEL, S, AREA, , 12, 13
NSLA, S, 1
SF, ALL, FSI        ! DEFINE COUPLE VIBRO-ACOUSTIC
FSI INTERFACE
```

```
ALLS
! READ ONE-WAY COUPLING CGNS FORMAT FILE
FLUREAD, , FFF_PRESSURE_F5, CGNS, , , , BOTH
ALLSEL
ECPCHG
FINISH

/SOLU
ANTYPE, HARM
HARF, 0.2, 10
NSUB, 20
ALLSEL
SOLVE
FINISH
```

Index

N

O

P

R

S

T

U

V